Looks Like We're RUNNING

An Amateur's Companion to
Becoming a Marathoner

Dustin Riedesel

Dedication

For my younger, reckless self. He's the guy who introduced me to marathon running.

More than once upon a time, Younger Self sat in a jail cell thinking he had ruined his life. I remember how much it all hurt him, the failure and the shame. But he kept going. He worked the steps. He started running, and he didn't stop. I'm proud of him for that.

Also, jail sucks, and Younger was really wallowing, so using the magic of dedication time travel, I'm telling him a joke:

"Why did the marathoner go to jail?"

Wait for it.

"For resisting a rest."

Table of Contents

Introduction:
The Chicago Marathon - October 13, 2019

"Okay, what am I doing here?"

This isn't a real question. It's just existential angst. That's all. What I'm actually doing is running mile eighteen of the 2019 Chicago Marathon. It's my first marathon, and my brain is just on a low, angsty simmer in spiritual synchronicity with the race's relentless pain.

"What am I doing *here*?"

I've been listening to music, relying on the tiny dopamine jolt that accompanies the beginning of a great song. It's the one thing that doesn't suck right now, an audible lifeline reminding me that the world is more than asphalt and torture. Then my AirPods die. They'll need at least twenty minutes to recharge. I put them back in their case, and the lid snaps closed like a coffin.

"What am I *doing* here?"

No one explained how far I'd have to go. Sure, the distance is precisely measured and mapped out in detail, but physical travel isn't really the point. Moving my body is simple. Right foot, left foot —I'm playing catch with inertia. I've been doing this for eighteen miles, and if my pace doesn't improve (which it won't), I'll keep playing catch for another eighty minutes. I know exactly where I'm going and what to do to get there, but I don't know how I'm going to do it.

If knowing what you don't know is the essence of wisdom, the next eighty minutes will be the wisest experience of my life.

"What am *I* doing here?"

Then I felt my first cramp. Right hamstring. It's not bad. I played college basketball, and when you've played an overtime game, ignored stretching, recovery, and sleep to stay up until 4:00 a.m. drinking fifteen beers, you know bad cramps. Imagine your hamstring is butter. Now put that butter in the freezer for hours and then stretch it like William Wallace at the end of *Braveheart*. By comparison, this first marathon cramp is more of a "whoopsie." I tell myself not to kick the right leg back too far. Three minutes later, my left hammy has a whoopsie. I decrease kick on that side too.

Seven miles to go. *What* am I doing here?

What I'm doing is keeping my legs straight, relying on my quads. I look more like a duck than a runner. I imagine my dehydrated muscles are beef jerky. Until now, I've been rotating Gatorade and water at stations. I'm double Gatorades the rest of the way. Flavor: Glacier Misery. I haven't stopped running since a porta-potty on mile four, but I'm desperate. I bend down and let my hammy jerky stretch. I have no idea if this is good for cramps, but it feels right. It feels like hope. And it is this decision that saves my race. Not because the cramps are eliminated—they'll come back—but because it buys me fifteen minutes. For fifteen minutes, I believe in my legs. *That* will carry me through mile twenty.

I don't know it, but my wife is trying to find me. She has Walter, our eight-month-old son in a bear-suit onesie, strapped to her chest. She's a visitor to Chicago, and she's been wandering through public transit and dense crowds for three hours. There are over fifty thousand runners, and I'm just one jogger in that haystack. If she's successful, and if I also see her, she'll get to cheer me on for ten seconds. It's a crazy amount of effort for something so small.

And she's done it. She's in front of me at mile twenty. And she starts jumping up and down, waving and screaming my name. And it's something like a miracle that I hear her, because my headphones are dead for only this moment. And we lock eyes, we smile, we wave. And in this moment, I'm proud of us both, and even if I can't articulate it fully yet, I can imagine that she's looking at me and seeing the man—the husband and father—that I always wished I could become. And maybe it is a temporary illusion, or maybe it's only a glimpse of a dream. It doesn't matter, because for those one hundred feet, all 26.2 miles are totally worth it.

What am I doing here? I don't really know, but I have six miles to go, and it looks like I'm running.

Looks Like We're Running
An Amateur's Companion to Becoming a Marathoner

Week 1
Get Out The Door

Katy Milkman is an award-winning professor of behavioral economics at the Wharton School of Business. She wrote a *Wall Street Journal* bestseller called *How to Change: The Science of Getting from Where You Are to Where You Want to Be.* The book offers a methodology to be applied to any lifestyle change, like quitting smoking, losing weight, keeping your house clean, or starting an exercise routine. I took notes, and I'll quickly adapt the first steps of that methodology to running.

Step One: Have a "Start Fresh" Date. This is a clear beginning, jumping into the pool with both feet. Once you're in, you're in. Milkman suggests a birthday or New Year's. For a marathon, I suggest doing the math backwards to calculate a starting point twenty weeks before the marathon. Monday is a great day for beginnings.

Step Two: Bundle in Fun. How do you make this new thing not suck? How do you make running enjoyable? To begin, you pair it with a treat. Run with friends. Finish runs at a coffee shop or a brewery. I like to save the podcasts and audiobooks I'm looking forward to for my long runs. For this particular marathon training, I purchased a Spotify subscription I'd been denying myself.

Step Three: Self-Imposed Restrictions: This is a commitment device. "I'm not allowed X until I run my miles." Not beginning your day until you've run is the most foolproof. Alcohol is a popular restriction. For me, the restful end of my day is TV or a movie with my wife. I can't sink into that couch until after the miles are logged.

Step Four: Cue-Based Plans. This is about manipulating your environment to create an outcome, and this is where I'll stop just writing Cliff Notes of another book. Because this is literally where the shoe rubber meets the road. The only cue you need is to get out the door. Put your shoes on and get out the door. Put your shoes out the night before, so you wake up, see them, put them on, and get out the door. Hell, put your shoes on the night before, sleep in them, and then they'll already be on your feet when you wake up and get out the door. Once you're in your shoes and out the door, you can't mess this up. I'll thank Professor Milkman in the "Special Thanks" section for infusing this chapter with some academic bona fides, but c'mon. This is running. Right foot, left foot. Simplest instructions in the world. Need a cue? Lean forward. A little further. You'll get it.

My dad is not a bestselling Wharton professor. He was, however, an award-winning (probably) paper salesman and little league baseball coach. He routinely said, "The main thing is to keep the main thing the main thing." Maybe 7 *Habits of Highly Effective People* said it first, but put the little circled "C" next to my dad. I can't imagine my dad outlining a plan for the most favorable psychological terrain on which to take his first, baby-soft steps, and I gotta say, I think his hypothetical lack of complexity is genius. Do you want to be a comedian? Get stage time. Do you want to be a writer? Write more. Do you want to touch your toes? Increase the time spent reaching for your toes. The most important ideas in life are simple and do not need much explanation. However, we must repeat these ideas over and over so that we don't take them for granted. Tell your spouse you love them. Tell your child you're proud to be their parent. Do not let the simple, important thing fade into the under-appreciated background like it's the air or the sun. This is true for anything you wish to prioritize, and it's true for running. Here's the simple and important idea: Get out the door.

In week one of training for the Disney Marathon, I run seventeen miles with a long run of seven miles. This long run is the shortest long run of training, but it still *feels* long. Other than the long run, no run this week takes longer than thirty-five minutes. For me, this is essential. It's not too hard, and there is no reason I can't find thirty-five minutes to run. I don't need to gear up or gas up. I only need to show up. I'm running in an old pair of Brooks Ghosts that have over seven hundred miles on their treads and double as lawn-mowing shoes. I wear basketball shorts and a purple TrailHeads hat I ran the Chicago Marathon in. That race was two years ago, and I haven't run consistently since. *Immaterial*, I tell myself. Just get started. Get out the door. Run. The rest of what we need is found on the trip, not prior to departure.

Keeping the main thing the main thing does not mean keeping it the only thing. There are many things about running that are not actually running. The first half of this book will discuss these things: an appropriate goal, a well-designed running schedule, the proper training shoes, rigorous cross-training, a beloved sleep routine, and more. What's the point of all this non-running talk? First off, this isn't a sex-ed book from the 1950s preaching abstinence. There's some cool shit out there. Enjoy it. Let's fool around with shoes and music and sleep and hydration. You're curious, and it's fun, and I'm sure you'll be responsible. Secondly, if you want to be the best runner you can be, you need to account for all the things, not just the main thing. If you can repeatedly get out the door, you will see significant improvement. Curving the grade to your talent, running consistently will change you from a below average runner to a B-plus or A-minus runner, but if you want those final few percentage points to become an A or an A+, you will need the other things.

But that's for later. It's Week 1. Just focus on the main thing. To get started, it's all you need.

Get out the door. Just move. Movement is the main thing for running, and it may be the main thing for life. There's a quote: "One run can change your day. Many runs can change your life." The more middle age invades, the more I appreciate my body's role in making me who I am. One of the most amazing and repeatable evidences of my body's role in our partnership can be observed when I'm stressed. Maybe I have a tough morning with the kids, or my job is pulling me in too many directions at once. Maybe I'm bummed about our country's latest political failure, or I have general anxiety about something I can't pinpoint. Whatever the stress, I can run for forty-five minutes and feel better. Nothing in the world has changed, and yet the world is a brighter, calmer, and less oppressive place. I used to tell myself I didn't have time to run. There was too much going on. Forty-five minutes was too high a cost. It isn't true. There is always time. It's a matter of prioritization. After the run, what I thought were four A-class priorities have been transformed into one A-class priority and three things that can be pushed or delegated. I'm healthier and happier, and the most important piece of work gets higher quality attention.

Get out the door. Just run, even if your life is already stress-free. A runner named Ronald Rook is famous for saying, "I don't run to add days to my life. I run to add life to my days." My take? I reject the false dichotomy. The older I get, the more I want to enjoy being old. I want more days and more life. I don't just want to know my grandkids, I want to play with them, like rolling on the ground type of play. That's years away, but running now helps make it possible. Smoking is terrible for you, right? I mean, smoking cigarettes feels like it's anti-running in a lot of ways. You stand still, you breath slow, and it's not oxygen filling your lungs and making you lightheaded. Here's a tidbit from Dr. Peter Attia, a researcher in human health and longevity. Did you know that doing easy cardio for forty-five minutes at least three times a week is more beneficial to your health than regular smoking is detrimental to your health?

The cardio correlates to a five times *decrease* in all-cause mortality. Smoking is a three times *increase*. To oversimplify, a smoker who exercises has a better chance at living longer than a non-smoker who doesn't exercise. So even if you don't need stress relief, running is a value add. Life is great! Let's live more of it!

Get out the door. It's good for your mind and body, but what about the rest of you? Olympic cyclist Kristin Armstrong said, "There is something magical about running; after a certain distance, it transcends the body. Then a bit further, it transcends the mind. A bit further yet, and what you have before you, laid bare, is the soul." You don't have to give Olympic effort for that result. Google "quotes for running," and you'll see that people don't talk about the running as much as they talk about themselves. When it comes to running, Oprah, Kelly Ripa, and Jon Hamm are just like us, and they not only talk about running as a vehicle for becoming better, but for becoming more of themselves. Jennifer Lopez, Cher, and Matthew McConaughey tell you running is the key to fun and happiness. Cameron Hanes, Haruki Marukami, David Goggins— they all tell you that running is way to know your limits and thereby know yourself. Who else do you need to hear from? Put on the shitty shoes you mow grass in and get out the door.

In closing this chapter, I'd like to give you what I think is an incredible gift. I've written a book within this book. That's right, it's a surprise two-for-one deal. This Russian nesting book is titled *The Self-Actualized Runner's Step-by-Step Guidebook for Living* and if I had any economic sense at all, I would have released it independently and become a *Wall Street Journal* bestseller like Professor Milkman. Here it is:

No Introduction. No foreword.

Step One: Start running.

Step Two: You've already taken it.

Step Three: Repeat steps one and two until you understand exactly who you are and why you do what you do.

Epilogue: Troubleshooting. Should runner become unable to run, take rest for no more than twenty-four hours and start again at step one. Add speed to taste.

Maybe you don't need *The Guidebook* to guide you, but I doubt it. If you don't use this one, you'll likely write your own in your head.

To balance all the "just do it" energy in this chapter, let me say this about completing week 1 of your training. It is a triumph. The first week is a noteworthy brick on the fortress of your identity. Take a beat on Sunday to pat yourself on the back. Eat a brownie or get a pedicure or whatever makes you feel like the royalty of your life. This week, you earned it. You got out the door. You ran. That's the main thing.

Week 0
Pre-Training: No One Wants to Run a Marathon

Wait, Week *Zero*? That's not real. Are we moving backwards? Stop. Listen up for a moment. Put your concerns on ice. Week zero has already happened. There's no action items, no pre-work. I just need to inject some narrative foundation into this book, and—in case some of our readers need to steel their resolve after a full week of running—I need to offer something more emotionally resonant than the "just do it" ethos of week one. Here we go:

What's your origin story? All heroes have one. When faced with uncertainty and fear, they tell themselves the story they've told themselves a thousand times before. They tell themselves why they do what they do, and they're rejuvenated to the cause. This story is their origin story. Truth is less important than effect. The story must inspire. The story must motivate. Spider-Man couldn't save his Uncle Ben, so he saves other people. Forrest Gump was born simple —some people would even say "slow"—but this origin inoculated Forrest from social fears; he lived without hesitation according to his convictions. Michael Jordan got cut from his high school team. Michael Jordan took that personally. Origin stories aren't about explaining the daily tasks that create a hero. Origin stories don't even explain who the hero becomes. Origin stories tell us why there's a hole in the hero's life that keeps them shoveling dirt, desperate to fill in the hole. What do they dream about? Michael Jordan wants to dominate others. Forrest Gump wants to belong. Spider-Man has more of a burden than a goal; he doesn't want to let anyone down. Now, these heroes—any heroes—do not need to be successful. Fulfillment is not the key to heroism. They are heroes because they understand what they want, and they pursue it courageously. So, what's *your* origin story? What story defines your desire?

This book is about running a marathon, and chances are good that you're a regular person, a "middle of the bell curve" type. Me too. We're only heroes in the "everyone's the hero of their own story" sense, but we still need an origin story. When one of us regular people tries to run a marathon, we face uncertainty and pain on a weekly basis. I won't say that running a marathon *is* heroic, but for us the effort will *feel* heroic, and sustaining that effort means telling ourselves a story we've told ourselves a thousand times before. Why am I doing this? Why did I ever want to run a marathon?

I've never given birth to a human child. From my perspective, that's the high-end of humanity's creative hierarchy. Nothing our species has built is as impressive as growing new life in a womb. To see the birth of a baby is witnessing to-scale the miracle of existence, and it is staggering. On the low-end of the creative hierarchy is one man. This man writing these words. Nice to meet you. The pleasure is inarguably mine. Also, my condolences. What's the low-end of creativity look like? Once, I wanted to enhance my style. I wanted to express my unique self via fashion. I decided the Chelsea Boot would do this. You've seen these. They come up a few inches above the ankle, and that ankle-coverage part of the boot is a U-shaped piece of elastic that allows the boot to be slipped on but also stay slim underneath a pair of pants. Why would that reflect the unique me? *PPbbhht*, you don't get it, man. I was giving birth to a new me, a cooler me. I compiled price differences, color preferences, and the cons of suede against the drab of leather. I kept a Google Images tab of "david beckham chelsea boot" in my browser at all times just in case my conviction waned. Finally, after six weeks of deliberation, I read a GQ article entitled, "How Chelsea Boots Turned Me into a Fashion Guy." The author described an experience exactly like my own, and recommended the suede, New Republic boot for the low price of ninety-nine dollars. I pulled the trigger. And holy shit! The boots worked! I wore them, and I forgot about the wishy-washy phase needed to generate courage. Self-esteem is the reputation you have with yourself, and these boots *did* give birth to a more confident, slightly cooler me.

Why am I telling you this? Because you should know this story you're about to embark on is not the work of an expert. Nor is this expedition guided by talent or genius, and I refuse to tell you otherwise. I'm not going to begin this relationship with a lie. I'm not a monster. No, I'm a man, and not just in the most traditional, reproductive sense of the word, but also in the low-end-of-species sense. I'm *only* a man, one who "fakes it" in hopes of "making it." Perhaps most informatively, I'm a man in the American-sitcom sense. White and educated with a good job, kids and a demanding schedule. I'm both successful and stupid as hell. I'll beat my chest near an expensive, wood-pellet grill and tell you I'm a *man*, but most of the significant women in my life have seen me insecure in my duties and thought, "He's just a *man*." They are accurate. At the heart of everything you are about to read is amateurism: a lack of experience counterbalanced by an abundance of love for the game. I know Chelsea boots aren't style, just like I know marathons aren't peace of mind. Amateurism is something you do purely because you have a feeling. That feeling is a doorway. You might be surprised at what you find on the other side.

How's that for an origin story? Hello, I'm Dustin: twenty-first century male, amateur runner, owner of confidence boots. Need more profile? Fine. I live in North Carolina. Our state motto is *Esse Quam Videri*: "To be rather than to seem." That seems like a pointless nugget, but sometimes things seem pointless until they're not. The difference is time. Can you try it? Can you stick with it long enough to find out? These things—you wear them, do them, or say them until a nugget chock-full o' points is the realest thing in existence.

I'm going to spoil something. This entire book is an origin story.

"To the confident man, every zoo is a petting zoo." I love that joke, not just because it's funny but because it's interesting. Comedian Bryan Callen says, "It's more important to be interesting than funny." We don't know the origin story of the man at the zoo —if he's successful or stupid as hell—but his confidence makes him interesting. When I sat down to give birth to chapter one of this how-to experience of running a marathon, I didn't have the proper how-to or the experience, but I wrote chapter one anyway. My logic was to write about the marathon like I trained for the marathon, and just getting started is the beginning. Art imitates life. Then again, you may have noticed this isn't chapter one. Only in hindsight did I realize that preparation for the Disney Marathon didn't start with the first week of training. I had multiple years of effort, including a prior marathon, to prepare me for the first week of Disney Marathon training. All of what's come before is my personal week zero. Experienced marathon runners may tell you that motivation is immaterial, that you run because that is what you do, and it is the habit of running that makes you a runner. They're not wrong but, if you're like me, you use an insecure emphasis to say, "I'm a *runner.*" You can hear hesitation in the word, how it's— *ugh*—vomited up. "I'm a r-*ugh*-nner." It sounds like hope struggling to breathe. Runners like us find the running hard and inconsistent and painful. We don't feel fast and steady. We're not beating our chest near the Ciele cap display telling people "I'm a *runner.*" Runners like us don't even know if we're pronouncing Ciele correctly on the audiobook version. Why didn't we choose different brand imagery? Dammit, we're filled with so much doubt. For runners like us, motivation is *very* material, so here we are in chapter zero. Before you ever take a step, you have to make choice. Do you want to run a marathon?

Wait! Don't stop reading. I know the answer to that question is obvious. No one *wants* to run a marathon.

Let's pull back. At the end of July 2021, my wife and I were on a family adventure. Most people take vacations, but if you have kids too young to speak coherent sentences, it's not a vacation. We're packed into a Florida beach house with twenty other family members and I ask my wife—her name is KT—I ask KT if we *really* want to sign up for the upcoming Disney Marathon in January. She says yes. I give The Mouse my money. The Mouse doesn't blink. I blink a little bit.

Let's pull further back. KT and I work in high-accountability tech companies. We have a mortgage, one rental property, young kids, friendships we work at, and some hobbies that consume too much time (like these words). What would make us decide to give up an entire waking day every month for five months? That's what it takes, by the way. If you're new, focused, and efficient, the time sacrifice of a marathon is roughly twenty-five hours a month. Why would we want to run a marathon?

The most honest answer is the simple: we just *wanted* to. But that can't be right. No one wants to run a marathon.

You want the extra-honesty behind that most honest answer and it's this: lies. We couldn't explain why we wanted to run a marathon, so we lied. We lied to ourselves about the time, effort, and pain. "It's on our bucket list," we lied, because we don't have a bucket list. We called it a dream, which is more acceptable than a lie, but all dreams are lies, really. The helpful dreams let us welcome pain and sacrifice earlier than later. When reality is born and the dream dies, maybe we can see clearly how much of it was lies. And hey, I'm glad we lied. I'm glad we dreamed. It takes bravery to chase dreams because dreams give birth to reality. That's the real justification for just *wanting* to do anything. Want is more beautiful than need specifically because it can turn a piece of a lie into the truth, a big dream into a little reality.

So I guess the extra-extra-honesty buried beneath the explanation of the most honest answer is this: We wanted to run a marathon because we wanted our lives to be different. There, I said it. Different how? We couldn't have told you. Thus, the dream. Thus, the lies.

This paragraph here, the very one you're reading now, was going to be filled with adoration for my wife. Unlike me, she has never run a marathon to prepare her for running a marathon. Also unlike me, she has given birth to not one, but two human children, and they are the two most spectacular children—nay, human beings—in the whole damn world. She did it with courage and grace, and when she had a moment to breathe and analyze the state of the strong, beautiful body that performed these feats, she said, "I'm going to be even stronger than before giving birth to those kids." Then she signed up for her first marathon ever and faced the grueling weeks that followed on a mission of capacity and resilience and progress. I signed up like two sports bras, extra supportive. Though I'm not a life-bringer like her, she is my motivation for running the Disney Marathon. I am the rock upon which a great woman stands all the taller…Only, immediately before writing this paragraph, I asked KT if she remembers why we signed up for the Disney Marathon, and it wasn't anything like that.

Apparently, when she was pregnant with Winnie, she said, "I'd like to run a marathon before I'm thirty-five."

I said, "Are you serious?"

She said, "I could be."

Why hello there, Origin Story, welcome to the planet. *Was* she serious?

She *could* be.

Dear reader, are you hooked? Isn't that enthralling? Why thirty-five? Seems arbitrary. It sounds like she just *wanted* to run a marathon, but no one wants to run a marathon. In 2015, *USA Today* published an article titled, "9 Reasons to Run a Marathon." Here's the list:

1. Achieving a goal
2. Building confidence
3. You'll test yourself
4. You'll gain more than you lose
5. Overcoming obstacles
6. Increasing fitness
7. Friendships
8. You'll explore new places
9. It will change you

If this had been a traditional ten-item list, number ten would have read: "You're turning thirty-five soon." I'm sure of this fact, as sure as I love my wife. Turning thirty-five is a meta-reason containing and yet simplifying all other reasons. Thirty-five is a milestone, and you're planting a flag. Embroidered on that flag is an equation, and it says 26.2 divided by thirty-five equals *it's not fucking over*. Running a marathon before turning thirty-five is transforming into a lioness and roaring, "I can have it all. Someone get me a Ciele cap!"

Are you starting to sense that nothing is happening here in week zero? Am I wasting your time? Where are the tips? Where do you get a good training plan? What kind of shoes do you need? Wouldn't it have taken less time to Google the pronunciation of "Ciele" than it took to write the joke about mispronouncing it? A real runner might tell you that nothing is happening because you're not running yet. They might be right, but they're not one of us. They're not a r-*ugh*-nner. They don't have to generate massive amounts of motivation to counterbalance their lack of experience, lack of talent, and lack of a general can-do attitude. They don't get it. "Just do it" is only good advice if you know what "it" is. So no, not much is happening here, and I'd like to offer you some grace. Grace as motivation.

Only one percent of the population has run a marathon. That means that ninety-nine percent of the population is here in chapter zero. They're not running a marathon. They all need a better reason to run. You may be one of them, looking for motivation, looking for a reason. You've heard a lot of other reasons. People tell you they're running because "I don't know" or because "It always sounded fun" or because "Just because." Then there are the unsaid reasons that people run, which are technically zero reasons, but also they are legion. People run because they're still single, or their dog died. Maybe they've been married too long. They got a promotion. Their house isn't big enough. They're not having sex. They're having too much sex. They just moved to a new city. Hell, it's cheaper than therapy.

If my examples tend to skew negative it's because I'm providing an accurate, representative sample of r-*ugh*-nners. People who don't run in four-hour races and have an otherwise great life don't often feel compelled to start running in four-hour races. Often, there's something wrong with life as it was before attempting the marathon. It can be a life-ender or a marriage-breaker, but it can also be anything that feels like resistance or stalling out. Stagnation is its own kind of life-ender. And this is where the real runners are right. You need to reach the end of week zero. You have to get moving. Why did my wife and I need to lie to ourselves? Why did we need a dream? The same reason anyone needs a dream. We needed something to chase.

For some people, stagnation feels like fog, a barrier between you and living. I think that's really why KT chose to run. Disney is her first marathon. She really is all the praiseworthy descriptions I wrote earlier, but *also*—God, let my wife read this with a forgiving heart—she was someone *else* in July of 2021. She was sleep-deprived and recovering from the routinely underrated trauma of passing an entire human body through her vaginal canal. She gave birth! This is the most amazing feat people can accomplish, but because everyone knows someone who has done it, we slap it with a couple months of "don't go to your job for a bit" and pretend we didn't just witness a miracle. Giving birth is kind of like how we rotate around a giant ball of nuclear fire that powers all life on this planet, but also we just sleep through sunrise like, "Welp, NBD." My wife gave birth twice in two years, and in this state of ho-hum PTSD, she decided a marathon was a good idea. She was going to run, damnit! But she wasn't going to say that our kids had set up roadblocks in her relationship with herself, so what did she have to say on the matter? She was turning thirty-five soon.

Then there's me. What was I lying about? I've already run one marathon. You read about it in the intro, remember? You were impressed by how I used the AirPods' death to evoke my own emotional state? You remember. Anyway, I don't know why I chose to run. I have a story I tell myself today, but I don't remember what the Dusty of the past told himself then. I think I was also in a fog. The three years prior had included surviving leukemia, going to rehab for alcohol addiction, and becoming a father. I didn't know who the hell I was. I was just trying to keep the train on the tracks. I was trying to be, I don't know, to be…

Ah! This is it! The nugget, chock-full o' points! *Esse Quam Videri.* You can't *seem* like a marathoner. You can only *be* a marathoner. That's what kept me going, the dream of being certain of myself, of being something solid. My body had failed to cancer. My mind had failed to substance abuse. But then I had a son, the first thing I'd ever loved unconditionally, and I sensed that a failure of the heart would break me beyond repair. I dreamed of integrity. *Esse Quam Videri.* Now, there are some things that *should* exist in a seeming way. The information on Google. The entertainment at Disney. That knowledge and those stories help us navigate our lives. But some things should exist in a solid way. They aren't *like* anything. These things are years of committed friendship or having kids or finishing the most difficult physical challenge of your life. These things aren't helpful metaphors. They are real and singular and foundational to your relationship with yourself. In such cases, you have experienced the journey or you have not, and there is only one way to know why you did what you did, and that way is to have done it!

I write a long letter to my children every year on their birthday. On Walter's first birthday, a few months after my first marathon, I wrote this: "How does a dad build a crib, install a car seat, support the neck, make formula, build a glider, change a diaper, give a sink bath, puree fruits and veggies, unpack a Pack 'n' Play, install pet gates, change a blowout diaper that is "Oh my God, it's everywhere," know when to take a temperature, call your mom to have her call the doctor, anchor nursery shelving, play patty-cake, sing "Sucker" by Jonas Brothers when mom's around, sing "Born to Run" by Bruce Springsteen when mom's in the shower, trick the dog into dropping your pacifier, make banana pancakes, or figure out what new game you'll be one hundred percent obsessed with for the next ten minutes? I just started doing these things, and I still don't know that I'm doing any of them "right," but I'm feeling a repetitive transition happening, that I'm taking activities from the ignorance pile and moving them into my skillset pile, that I'm transitioning humility towards pride, and maybe, just maybe, if I can keep this up for another couple of decades, maybe you'll be able to tell people you had a great dad."

I wrote that three months after the Chicago Marathon. *Keep going.* That's what my first marathon taught me. If I have the means to move my body a mile, then I can move it for 26.2 of them. And why would I do such a thing? The answer is at the finish line.

But why am I running this second marathon? I believe running has more to teach me. I've said repeatedly that no one want to run a marathon. That's partially a joke. What's not a joke is that everyone who runs a marathon *wants*. The marathon is for those who want to be more or be better or just be different. Mostly, they want answers about what they are *really* made of. My life has new responsibilities since the first marathon. I have a daughter. I've been promoted to leadership at work. Writing won't leave me alone. The first marathon taught me that answers were at the finish line, and I'm running this second marathon because I've recently learned that the finish line is farther away than I thought.

If you are able to complete your first marathon—or achieve that new PR—the answers you will receive about yourself are not trivial. You will realize that you are less anxious and less afraid and generally stronger than you previously knew. You will see yourself more clearly and, just as important, you will *know* that you see yourself more clearly. And you know what that sounds like to me? That sounds like a damn good origin story.

Week 2
The Goal is Success

Here's my entire history of organized races prior to signing up for the 2022 Disney Marathon.

April 2018: Rock 'N' Roll 5K in Raleigh, NC - 00:23:14
June 2018: Rock 'N' Roll Half Marathon in San Diego - 1:59:53
October 2019: Chicago Marathon - 4:23:32

Here's the thing about that timeline. Four months before the first 5K, I'd never run farther than three consecutive miles in my life.

Here's another thing about that timeline. I received a final dose of chemotherapy only seven months before that 5K. I had leukemia. It still feels weird to say this, but it's no hyperbole whatsoever. Cancer nearly killed me. I spent thirty-three days in the hospital followed by ten months of chemotherapy. The toll of such an experience is significant, and it isn't just physical. The heart and mind are also afflicted, but that damage is more subversive, and there are no health insurances, doctors, or nurses with a medical miracle to piece you back together. In that ten months of chemo, I stayed home from work drinking way too much (and getting fat) while my new wife went off to work. I'd never felt so lucky, and not in the good way. I was manic with self-pity for how little I'd earned my life. I'd gleefully talk to people about how fortunate I felt to survive, but when I was alone, there was a depression rising up around me like a slowly filling bathtub. Twice I can remember during chemo, I had drunk dialed friends and was crying to them on the phone when

KT showed up. She should have been at work, but the friend keeping me on the line had also texted her, fearing I was in danger of hurting myself. I don't think I was ever *really* suicidal, but that's something where in denying it, well, one doth protest too much. Bottom line, I was not in a good place.

Honoring my midwestern heritage, I acted like everything was fine and just pressed on. The chemo wrapped. They gave me a fun little purple-heart certificate, and then I found twenty dollars. What's next? I thought the answer was trying to do everything, to be everything. *Carpe diem*! I was a cancer survivor, damnit! I owed, something? I owed—I don't know—I owed life! I was like Tony Soprano in season five, but without the safety net of crime, murder, and adultery to ease back into. I had to get back to work. So I returned to my Fortune 100 job. I got involved with the Leukemia & Lymphoma Society. I wrote and published a book about the millennial generation (because that book had nothing to do with what I was actually going through, I remember it as a monument to numbing). I socialized in the evenings, and I woke up early in the mornings to work out. And when New Year's of January 2018 showed up, it wasn't a milestone. It was a challenge. My first year cancer-free. I would press harder. I made a resolution to get in the best shape of my life. I dieted to counteract the drinking and weight gain. I started running and scheduled the 5K and the San Diego Half, but also, I wanted more life, figuratively and literally. I planned a vacation to Hawaii, and KT and I began trying for kids. 2018 was going to be epic.

Spoiler: 2018 was not epic. One of the reasons I'm writing *Looks Like We're Running* on top of *The Self-Actualized Runner's Guidebook for Living* is because the steps outlined in *The Guidebook* proved insufficient for my needs. I know! I'm shocked too, but it's true. Two thousand eighteen was a fucking grind, and not in the cutesy way successful people joke about, "Rise and grind, get that bread." No, it was a grind in the way hardly anyone ever talks about because of shame.

Goals. That's what I want to talk about, and not in the Tony Robbins way. Self-help books and coaches tend to talk about goals like a commodity. Do you have enough goals? Are your goals big enough? What is your goal worth to you? Relax. This is only week 2 of training. Let's let the giant within stay there for now. Goals aren't commodities. Goals are relationships. Measure less. Relate more. If you build them correctly, goals are friendships you create with yourself.

Have you ever thought deeply about friendship? I don't mean analyzing the people you call "friends" like taking a relational inventory (although that sounds helpful too). I mean thinking about what makes *you* a friend to someone else. And what do *you* get out of that friendship? Have you examined this concept, having friends, or did it walk through the TSA of your life on one of those utterly inexplicable times where the shoes stay on? Don't look the gift horse in the mouth! You understand that phrase. We all do. So I don't blame you if you just gathered your friendships and kept the line moving, but let's analyze friendship *now*.

Friendship is a give and take. Good friends give you a lot. Whether through effort or charisma, they give you a sense of style, musical taste, career options, emotional support and forgiveness. Other stuff? Sure. The experience is dynamic and complex, and over time, this experience shapes your identity. Bad friends—you guessed it—take a lot. They take your time, dismiss your effort, bleed your support, and beg your forgiveness. This experience also shapes your identity. But what is your responsibility in these exchanges? What do *you* give? What do *you* take?

Sorry for all the questions. This isn't a riddle. I'll give you the answer. Friendships don't measure. Friendships relate. If you think about the five best friendships throughout your lifetime, they probably weren't about how much you gave or how much you took. They were about balance, and a trust that the balance was always paid off because the other side of the friendship appreciated all that was given and resented nothing that was taken. This is the answer to many relationships. Measure less, relate more. There is give and take, but not in the sense of debit and credit. The give and take is simply tension, the slack or taut of an enduring connection. Maintain this connection long enough, and it will shape your identity.

The tension of friendship is when you don't approve of the other person's behavior. Perhaps you feel compelled to say something, to stage an intervention, or to simply ignore the other person until they correct the behavior. Put anything under tension for enough time, and it will break. Sometimes the snapping point is hard to define, but you can always recognize the break in hindsight. When a friendship has lost all ability to shape your identity, it is broken.

In week two of training for the Disney Marathon, I run nineteen miles with a long run of eight miles. I'm focusing on good form and building routine. I'm spending as much time lifting and doing yoga as I am running. Is that a good plan? I don't know. This sub-four-hour goal is still a new friendship. We're still getting to know each other. I'm still more of a weight room guy than a running guy, but as we spend some time together, I'm sure I'll change.

Goals are friendships we create with ourselves, the abstract filters we use to purify our identity. Goals are about evolution, not achievement. You can choose to think of goals as achievements, and I suppose that would make goals more like a business partner you create with yourself. No one ever writes "business partners" on the short list of relationships that define their identity. But friends? They're here for the journey, not the outcome. Since this is a book about amateurs running a marathon, we'll talk about goals in that framework. Can you commit to a running goal? Can you give to running and take from running? Can you let running shape you? Bottom line: can you and running become good friends?

Before you answer that, let's zoom back. Here's a good mantra, a big-picture mantra for all walks of life: The only goal is success. You'll have hundreds of goals in life, but they're all really sub-goals of the only goal: success. It's a lot like in sports, how "the goal" is literally scoring a goal, but scoring a goal is actually just a sub-goal of winning the game, and winning the game is a sub-goal of winning a championship. Once you recognize this nesting-doll structure of all goals, you'll want to adjust how you build your training plan and layer your ideas of success.

Here's what I mean. I ran the Chicago Marathon in 4:23:32, and there were no layers to that goal. The dreamlike pride I felt seeing my family at mile twenty disappeared as soon as KT and Walter were out of sight. The next hour was filled with cramps, aches, and strangers saying platitudes like, "You got this," as they slogged past my sloggier slog. I crossed the finish line in 23,336[th] place, just missing the podium. I appeased my millennial heart with a participation medal which unironically read, "Finisher." Then an overwhelming sense of satisfaction rolled through my body and into my fingers as I texted KT, "That was worth it." I knew instantly that it was not my last marathon. Running and I weren't trying to achieve something. Running and I were going to hang out. My new friend had layers, and I needed to appreciate running for better and worse. In his book, 26 Marathons, the great, American marathoner Meb Keflezighi talks about cascading goals. An audacious "A Goal" that is achievable if you run your best race. A "B Goal" that would make you feel satisfied about the work you put into training. Finally, a "C Goal" that keeps you motivated even when everything has gone tits up (as they say). I like this structure quite a bit, and for my Disney Marathon, my A Goal is running a sub-four-hour marathon, shaving almost a minute per mile off my Chicago time of 4:23:32. My B Goal is running under that Chicago time to achieve a new PR. My C Goal—the tits-up scenario—is finishing, which I'll feel way better about than quitting. There is a D Goal, which is just a personal knowledge that I did my best, but I don't think about it much. Goals A through C exist to ensure Goal D is automatic even if the most uppity tits occur.

If this is your first marathon, then I wouldn't worry about which way the tits are facing—now that I've said "tits" so much, I regret the analogy. Anyway, finishing is great. Having the experience is great. I'm not being facetious. Ask anyone you know. Completion feels good. Okay, that *was* facetious—when did this chapter get so horny?—but it's also true. Running 26.2 miles for the very first time needs no additional qualifiers. In fact, unless you've had a serious running background like college cross country or something, then aiming for an audacious time could put too much stress on your training and lead to injury.

Sidebar: I'll say this as clearly as possible. Injury is the worst possible outcome of training. This will come up again later, but let it sink in now. When the goal is success, injury is the worst possible outcome of training. Alright, back to goals.

My wife's goal is to finish (Agh! Really regretting those "completion" jokes now, AREN'T I?). She's never finished *a marathon* before. I don't know if she'll feel the need to run a second marathon. Statistically, most marathoners don't run a second time. But when she's crossed the finish line, she will know that she's capable, resilient, and unafraid. *That* is success.

This will be hard for competitive people to hear, but comparison is silly. The goal is only helpful because it is specific to the athlete. Stretching the definition of athlete to talk in the first person: My A Goal is to beat me. My B Goal is to beat me. My C Goal is to beat me. I am my competition, running against my friend, the old version of me who helped me get here. You get it. This is not a difficult intellectual exercise. But ego is the enemy. Right now, when you're running nineteen-mile weeks and eight-mile long runs, don't be tempted to make a big, hairy, audacious goal. What's the point? Are you trying to finish 21,112[th] at the Chicago Marathon? Hey, nothing wrong with that, assuming you've taken accurate stock of yourself. But long-distance running is a long-term relationship. Building capacity and speed takes months. Building exceptional capacity and speed takes years. If you're creating a goal by looking at what others are capable of, then your goal is not going to help you tailor a training plan that will make you the best you can be.

When thinking of your personal goals, know that it's not the race that will drive you crazy. It's the training. An insane goal requires crazy commitment: money for the best gear, training time that cuts into your workday, your spouse's emotional and domestic support as you disappear for those long runs, and forgiveness from all involved as your personality is replaced by an odometer. Professional runners are that crazy, but their insanity is redeemed by dollar bills. If an amateur tries that, well, we're not *runners*. We only look like we're running. My suggestion is to be practical when you pick a goal, because a goal's purpose is to inspire a training plan. Our training plans are about balance. If we can manage our time, purchase discount gear, tend to our careers and families, then the training plan that results from all that conscientious effort has the highest likelihood of success. After all, shaving ten minutes off your PR is far less satisfying after getting fired. The medal that commemorates your sub-four-hour marathon is less fun to look at when it reminds your spouse that you're simply not around that much.

When you remove all the ornamentation and metrics we use to judge each other, success boils down to only one thing: peace of mind. You have it, or you don't. It is my experience that a specific goal, like running, requiring incremental effort over a set period of time is likely to give you greater peace of mind. It is also my experience that pursuing that same goal while ignoring the factors external to the goal can lead to despair.

Just something worth considering.

Alright, back to 2018. I'll keep this short and get us into next week. You don't want to hear about my 2018, not really. Here's the Cliff Notes. I was running hard and drinking harder. More than once, I woke up on whichever floor of the house I passed out on the night before. I changed clothes and went running before sunrise and before my wife woke up. In some unexplored corner of my mind, I had decided that if I ran, if I did my job well, if I *looked like* I had it all together, then I *did* have it all together. I thought success was an achievement.

It's obvious now that there's no peace of mind in drinking until midnight and running before 6:00 a.m., but I refused to look at my pain back then. Perhaps willful ignorance was a helpful defense for pushing through cancer and chemo. KT had also just miscarried in her first pregnancy, and maybe I was afraid that being present for her pain would be the saddest I've ever felt because I'd never loved like that or wanted something for someone so much. Maybe those are all bullshit excuses because I was really just an addict failing to fix himself. I don't *really* know. The "why" seems less important now anyway. I know that my mind refused to analyze the pain in my heart, and their conflict was torturing my body. The mind, heart, and body are the three pillars of being human, and I was failing to stand up any one of them.

After some heartbreaking chaos I won't punish myself with here, the pain couldn't be ignored. I took medical leave from work and did thirty days of rehab with a company called Two Dreams on the Outer Banks of North Carolina. In an immersive introduction to recovery, I began befriending the ugliest side of myself—a side I hid behind a false identity. I spent all my time around other addicts, in group therapy, at AA meetings, in one-on-one sessions with an addict turned licensed clinical addiction specialist. The huckleberry of this false-identity assassination was a letter from my wife that said bluntly all the worst things I'd ever done to her and myself. Impossibly, she signed it, "I love you so much."

The rehab felt long and terrible but also rewarding. I read novels by Jonathan Franzen and Nathan Hill. I wrote the first outline of my own novel. The other clients, all as broken as me, were encouraging. We played games and had some laughs. By the second week, as long as I was back in time for house breakfast, I was allowed to go running on the beach as the sun rose. The sand beneath my feet was more unsteady than the road, but that felt like the exact right place to be. I would do three miles every morning, and as the sky brightened into melting sherbet, I began to create a new goal, a new friend to help me become better. I would write and run. Those efforts could purify my mind and body, but what about my heart?

KT also sent me nice letters with words that didn't eviscerate my self-image but reminded me that there was good in me too. My vision was blurry, but she saw the good clearly enough, and her descriptions gave me hope. She called me a couple weeks before my stay was over to let me know she was pregnant. I couldn't believe it. Matters of the heart often require some luck, and it felt like we were both getting some when we needed it most. Then, two days before I was set to leave rehab, I got another call.

She had miscarried again.

Was she sure?

Ninety-five percent. She'd go to the doctor in a couple days for medicine to help pass everything.

I was so sorry, but what was there to say?

Did I need to stay longer to deal with it?

I said I was fine. I ran the next morning, and as I ran, I thought about "earning the sunrise," and how you had to give to the miles before they gave back. "Forgiveness" means to give before anything is owed. Maybe that's how I could heal the heart. KT was asking about my well-being when she was about to lose another child.

Maybe she needed me as much as I needed her. So that was the third pillar. I would pour into her and let the effort purify my heart. It would work. It had to work. The truth is, I had no idea if I would be okay, but I had a desire and a shitload of slogans, so keep it simple, stupid. One day at a time! I didn't need some twenty-year plan weighing me down. KT pulled up. I got in the car, and she handed me the most beautiful thing I've ever seen in my entire life. It was a strip of sonogram photos. She hadn't miscarried after all.

The day I walked out of rehab was the very first time I saw my son, and I recognized the goal immediately. Body and mind were accounted for, and now, here was my brand-new heart, beating inside the body of the woman I loved.

One year later, I ran by KT and our son at mile twenty of a race I finished in 23,336th place, successful as hell.

Week 3
The Best Advice: How to Build Your Training Plan

Amateur running has long been buttressed by the supposition that running farther, faster, and more often is the key to running better, but there is no one size fits all. Creating the best training plan for you is a dynamic and complex effort that requires speed work, longer easy runs, proper frequency for recovery, and attentive cross-training to build aerobic capacity and overall speed while limiting risk of injury. The failure to prepare such a plan is the same as a plan to fail—pfft!

GTFO. What am I, a coach?

The best writing advice I've ever received—and still receive repeatedly, not that I understand why—is to use classic, one-three-one structure. Introduction with a thesis statement, three body paragraphs, conclusion. Tell 'em what you'll tell 'em. Tell 'em. Tell 'em what you told 'em. The ol' one-two-three that's really the ol' one, one again, and once more. It's fool-proof. Militaristic wordsmithing to execute the mission objective. Yes, *structure* is certainly the best advice, and I'll be sure to use it the moment I run out of toilet paper! That may not be a creative joke, but we covered this in chapter zero. I'm not a creative person. I'm the kind of person who shits on the best advice.

Don't be like me. You don't have to see structure like I do, all straight-jackety. You know what it is for me? Structure makes everything feel like "have to." I *have* to run today. I *have* to do core work. I *have* to make it through one chapter without poop or tits or generally sophomoric behavior. I hate "have to." Always will, if I have to guess. Which I don't. I'm a "gets to" guy, even to my detriment. I'm only happy when I *get* to run, or when I *get* to slip in SAT vocab to juxtapose all the poop. This is why, to my own detriment, I didn't hire a coach or pay for a training plan. I didn't want to have to do anything.

So how should you structure your training plan? You shouldn't. You should hire a coach. The best coach of all time is Mickey Goldmill. He turned a bum from Philadelphia into Rocky Balboa. No real-life coach can match him. His training methods include chasing chickens, punching frozen meat, abstinence, and a salmonella diet. Mickey knows all the stuff Rocky doesn't. He creates accountability and makes the work more fun. He says stuff like, "You're gonna eat lightning and crap thunder!" But most importantly, Mickey fights for Rocky when Rocky won't fight for himself. The goal is functionally a relationship with a version of yourself you have yet to achieve. A good coach has all the knowledge, pain and experience to believe in that version of you even in the toughest moments of training. A coach gives you structure for the way forward, but they also act as a defense against your greatest enemy: yourself. The best advice to structure your training plan is to get a coach.

The second-best advice is to pay for a customized training plan built specifically to your goals and abilities. It's less accountable but more affordable.

But what if you're the kind of person who will spend one hundred hours training but not spend one hundred dollars planning. Then you're the kind of person who shits on the best advice. Even worse, you're the kind of person who knows you're this kind of person. It's okay. We're all hypocrites sometimes, and there is good news for those of us who refuse the best advice. We get better too. Our progress is slower and more painful than those who get help, but if we schedule that race and work our erratic, unstructured ass off to get there, we get better too.

In week three of training for the Disney Marathon, I run twenty-two miles with a long run of eight miles. Highlight of the week is a new training shoe, the Saucony Endorphin Speed 2. It's the first running shoe I've trained in that isn't the Brooks Ghost model, and it feels like I'm on springs. I match my 5K PR during my first tempo run in the shoes. It's gotta be the shoes! I agonized for weeks over articles and videos comparing dozens of trainers. Then I ran in the Speed. Sometimes, no matter how well a case is made, you have to feel it for yourself. The problem with this new feeling is that it is excellent. Like any addict, I know my budget is a feeble defense against recreating good feelings.

The difference between a structure and a plan is just something I made up. When asked if he was worried about Evander Holyfield's fight plan, Mike Tyson said, "Everyone has a plan until they get punched in the mouth." To run for twenty weeks and finish a marathon is difficult. A lot can go wrong. How would I guard my plan against a punch in the mouth? Structure is sturdier in mind. It's personalized to my life, and it's less about driving the outcome than it is about navigating the obstacles. When talking about human happiness, a well-structured life creates routines of improvement over routines of comfort. All you have to do is show up for the right routines and positive outcomes will create themselves. I believe this is true in the arc of life and in the minutia of endeavor. You can create routines of improvement in running. To do so, you must structure a life that can do it even when the punches are telling you that you can't do it. You need a structure that defends the running against the excuses. Punches, obstacles, excuses: they're all the same thing. And the big ones usually come in the form of time, money, knowledge, experience, luck, and grit.

Time. You don't have it, and the miles take as long as they take. Structure an abundance of time to plan, prepare, and execute those miles. Also to recover. You probably need to cut some other things out.

Money. As we start talking about diet and recovery, the money escalates quickly. There can be travel costs and race fees. If you don't have money, the punches of bad luck, ignorance, and inexperience will hurt worse. While the cost of running gear is minimal when contrasted with efforts like cycling and CrossFit, proper gear is still expensive. I'll talk about how to prioritize in the next chapter.

Knowledge. Your brain can't think you into shape, but it sure as hell can think you out of shape. This is what Chapter One was all about. Don't overthink it. "I don't know how" is an unacceptable excuse. You know how to run. You know how to recover (it's called not running). You know how to run farther than you did two days ago. If you're concerned about not knowing the details — training zones, carb-loading, electrolyte ratios, do you run slightly faster after a fart? — well, you can hire a coach or learn it the old-fashioned way, which is…

Experience. Ah, the partner of wisdom. There is no substitute. The difference between knowledge and experience is the difference between buying a suit off the rack and having one custom-cut and tailored to your exact dimensions. Experience is bespoke! With experience, you will know what works for you. Without it, you pay an extra tax spending more time, money, grit, and knowledge until you've become experienced. It's the most valuable asset you can possess and there's only one way to get it.

Luck. It is everything you can't control. Injury, weather, global pandemics, local track availability, talent, and everything else. Any structure that doesn't acknowledge the role of luck puts your mindset at risk. Bad luck can easily destroy an A Goal, and if you can't see luck's role, you may despair and put your B Goal or C Goal at risk as well.

Grit. A good structure is designed to create pain. A good structure makes demands when you have excuses. Ninety percent of the time, the only way out is through.

The next few weeks of this book build structure in this order:

- Gear (this is mostly about money)
- Time, mileage, and running (time, knowledge, grit)
- Cross-training and mobility (luck, grit, experience)
- Nutrition and hydration (luck, money, knowledge)
- Sleep and recovery (time, luck, grit, experience)

After all that, we're going to be deeper into the training and deep into the shit. That's the last thing about structures. They're built to be obsolete. We outgrow them. The structure provides space while we adjust our perception of what is difficult. Eventually, we will outgrow the structure. Trust me, we will eventually be able to stop worrying about "how to do this" and we will just be doing it. That's when we're done with all the advice; we're just running, moving forward. That's where I'd prefer to be anyway, a place where the best advice is to stop wiping my ass and get to work.

Week 4
Just Do It: All You Need Are Shoes and Socks and Something to Cover Your Junk and Eventually a Water Bottle and Probably a Cell Phone or a Running Watch and Some Headphones Are a Nice-to-Have

Just do it.

Those three words are the most brilliant sales pitch of my lifetime. Nike. Those fucking guys. People, rather. No need to discredit the smarmy marketing acumen held by all genders. Those fucking people. It's only week 4 but I'm going to spend over three hundred dollars with Nike before this training plan is finished, and before you ask, yeah, I'm hitting the sales and buying at clearance. Ask me how much I *saved*.

Just do it.

Remember the movie *What Women Want* starring Helen Hunt and Judy Greer—that girl is in everything—and Mel Gibson was there too. Actually, this is mostly a Mel joint; ironic, considering what women want from him now, which is not much. Hey, looks like we're judging. In the movie, Mel plays an advertising executive who gains the supernatural ability to read women's minds. How did he gain this troublesome power? He was shaving his legs, unclogging his pores, and blow-drying his hair all at the same time. Like. A. Female. He slips and falls into the bathtub where the hair dryer electrocutes him into a telepathic demigod. Stranger things have *happened*? Just go with it. How does Mel use this troublesome power? He starts by having sex with Marisa Tomei. Hell yeah. Then he steals intellectual property from Helen Hunt. Yahtzee! This guy is on a roll (Mel does eventually make amends with the women in his life, including coming through for his daughter in the clutch. He's not a monster. He's just a *man*).

Back to the plot: The pilfered intellectual property is an ad campaign to land Nike. Let me say that name again: Nike! More specifically, the "women's running division" which is probably how Nike segments its business entities. Despite all the shots I've just taken at both Mel Gibson and the larger plot of *What Women Want*, watching this fictional ad campaign for the first time was legitimately compelling, and dare I say it? Will I say it? Just say it. This ad campaign was insightful. I was fifteen, and I did not know what women wanted, and damnit if Mel Gibson narrating Helen Hunt's IP didn't tell me something about the dueling pressures of feminine expectations and free self-expression. The ad goes like this:

You don't stand in front of a mirror before a run...
and wonder what the road will think of your outfit.
You don't have to listen to its jokes and pretend they're funny.
It would not be easier to run if you dressed sexier.
The road doesn't notice if you're not wearing lipstick.
It does not care how old you are.
You do not feel uncomfortable...
Because you make more money than the road.
And you can call on the road whenever you feel like it,
Whether it's been a day... or even a couple of hours since your last date.
The only thing the road cares about...is that you pay it a visit once in a while.
Nike.
No games.
Just sport.

Could a shoe do all that? That's what fifteen-year-old me was thinking. Nike was a shoe company. I didn't understand how brands incepted a seed identity into a person's brain with words and imagery, then watered it for years on end until it germinated two decades later in a three hundred dollar pre-marathon spending bonanza. I thought the process was more like, "Oh, I like that commercial. When the soles of my current shoes have literal holes in them, I will consider a Nike shoe as a replacement." But why am I talking about shoes? The ad didn't mention a shoe. It didn't say anything at all. It said, "No games, just sport."

For context, *What Women Want* came out in May of 2000. The "Just Do It." ad campaign ran from 1988-1998, so "Just sport" wasn't a huge creative leap for the folks who figured out the bathtub-telepathy connection. Still, they nailed it. They captured the vague specificity that "Just Do It." commanded. "Just Do It." isn't a picture; it's a mirror. "Just Do It." isn't a plan; it's a philosophy. It's a way of life. It's your life, or, it *can* be your life if you can just get started. Get out the door. Get on the road. The rest of what you need is found on the trip, not prior to departure.

In week four of training for the Disney Marathon, I run twenty-four miles with a long run of seven miles. Even though my mileage increases, I count it as a deload week by decreasing the long run and keeping the easy runs easy. I was planning to run twenty-two miles but messed up the math. Whatever. It's fine. The seven-mile run was the highlight. It's September 11th, and I'm going to run laps around the North Carolina state capitol, where there are monuments to those who served in Vietnam and World War I. I was a sophomore in high school when 9/11 happened. My brother was a freshman at the Air Force Academy at the time, and I was afraid they were going to send him to war. My grandpa was a veteran of war. Maybe I considered the military, but it's more honest to say I was always too scared to consider the military. The monuments give off an atmosphere. It's easier to feel grateful for men like my grandpa and my brother, men who weren't too scared. I like to think my grandpa knew me. My brother knows me. They probably saw my fear, and they probably saw it in a lot of their fellow Americans. I like to think those men chose what they chose specifically so someone like me can happily run his ass off in a new pair of shoes. My gratitude is self-serving, but it's sincere. One warm-up mile followed by a fast five-miler followed by a cool-down mile. I run the five miles in thirty-eight minutes even, a 7:35/ mile pace. I'm feeling good! Maybe it's the new shoes? Maybe I've underrated the value of good gear? Feels that way.

Let me put my cards on the table. In the past year, I have acquired a lot of running gear. Some of it as gifts. Most of it is me spending my US dollars like a happy, American consumer. Here's the list of prices without tax or shipping:

Apple Watch SE - $350
Saucony Endorphin Speed 2 - $160
Saucony Triumph - $99
Nike ZoomX Vaporfly Next 2% - $200
Under Armour SpeedPocket 5" Short - $38
Starter 3" Run Short - $20
Balega Blister Resist Quarter Sock - $17
Rogue Runner Cap x2 - $50
Nike Dri-Fit Rise 365 Tank Top - $38
Nathan Speeddraw Insulated Water Bottle x2 - $75
Goodr Sunglasses - $25
Body Glide - $10
R5 Gore-Tex Infinium Jacket - $270
Total: $1,352

The jacket is a truly indefensible purchase, and I love it. Tattoo

"Infinium" on my butt cheeks. No regrets. I'm not going to mention my wife's running gear expenses except to say they were lower than mine. Good items not on this list include running tights and wireless headphones, both of which I already owned. Should you spend all this money? Probably not, but just do it. If this all seems expensive to you, I'll remind you that you're already into this running hobby for upwards of twenty dollars after buying this book. In poker terms, you're basically pot committed.

In all seriousness, finding gear to buy solves itself. If running blossoms for you as it has for me, you'll create spending justifications. You'll look at a $250 pair of shoes that makes you two percent faster and you'll just do it. This chapter isn't a consumer's guide. It's more of an obvious warning. Running is an industry supported by a global community. It's not a cult; it's a culture, and cultures are environments of growth, not just for your health and discipline, but for more unsavory habits too, like consumerism. My first piece of advice on buying gear is the same as my first piece of advice for running a race: Don't come out too hot. Don't feel pressured by those running around you. Don't just do it. Know yourself and run at your own pace. The only person you're in competition with is yourself.

If you are truly starting from scratch, then here's my approach on big-ticket items.

Shoes: Go to a local running store and talk to the staff. Here in Raleigh we have a shop called Runologie, owned and operated by a legit community of runners. Tell the staff about your background, what you're trying to achieve. These folks have run the miles, and they want what's best for your feet and body. They're not building a global empire. They're just legitimate fans of the running experience, and they create friends by sharing what they love. It's your best bet to get good advice on what shoe will be good for you, and you might even make a friend out of it. Most local shops have good running clubs.

If you don't have a local store, online research can guide you. I've done individual research to choose shoes from Brooks, Saucony, Asics, and Nike, and they have all been satisfying. These companies do such a great job with their products these days that your margin for error in shoe selection is very forgiving.

If you have a lot of money or passion, consider a multi-shoe rotation. I use a soft, supportive shoe for the long and easy runs (the Triumph), a faster trainer for my speed work (the Endorphin Speed 2), and an indulgent race-day shoe that makes me feel special (the infamous Nike Vaporfly). I do this mostly for personal preference, but also because recent studies (such as one published in the *Scandinavian Journal of Medicine & Science in Sports*) suggest that a shoe rotation leads to a significant decrease in the likelihood of injury. This makes a lot of sense considering that most running injuries come from repeating the same movements and impacts thousands of times. Variation is relief. We'll cover this more in the recovery chapter.

Running Watch: The advice is simple. Get one! I've used a FitBit in the past, currently use an Apple Watch, and have a lot of friends who rave about the Garmin offerings. For us amateurs, any of these venerable brands will be super pleasing. Their GPS is reliable, they have plenty of music storage, and—most important—they look badass. Garmin has my favorite aesthetics, but in each instance, wearing a running watch instead of a gaudy—dare I say try-hard—fashion-first timepiece is a style upgrade that says, "I'm about the work. I'm about function. I'm about substance." It's hard for someone like me to trade money for wrist decor that tells people I have a lot of money, so maybe you won't vibe with this message, but here it is: The deepest essence of "cool" is not giving a shit about anything except the things you *really* give a shit about. Unless you're James Bond obscuring your deep sense of mission and gadgetry with the trappings of an Omega, the running watch is way cooler than the style watch.

And the function!? Wow, don't get me started. Seriously. I don't want to talk about this, and I don't need to. The research for your watch purchase will bombard you with functionality. Battery life, heart rate tracker, pulse oximeter, sleep tracking, terrain insights, app integrations, blah blah blah. The only essentials in my opinion are heart rate, solid GPS, and accurate time. Those are important to your training, so you should *definitely* invest in a watch. Which one is your call. The watch doesn't support your run and health like a shoe, so the details are mostly preference.

Almost everything else in the "gear" category is preference. Everything but the shoes has marginal to no importance in your performance. Don't be fooled by oxygenated spandex, zero-gravity socks, or sunglasses that visualize excellence. Sure, you need warm clothes to run in freezing weather, and it's probably best to not do your speedwork in Wrangler's, but the gear doesn't get you fitter. You get you fitter. I love the gear. I love wearing my hobby into my identity. But Helen Hunt via Mel Gibson was right. The road doesn't care what you're wearing. Nike was right (maybe self-serving, but probably sincere). Even if you never give Nike a dime, you should remember what Nike was right about. The only way to improve is to get out there and run.

Just do it.

Week 5
Run Longer or Faster

At their core, great ideas are simple. Treat others as you want to be treated. What doesn't kill you makes you stronger. Newton's three laws of motion are all simple and profound. Money as a concept—a universal placeholder of value—is simple and great. I'd argue that an idea can't be great unless it is simple. Sure, you can have a complex thought or experience that is deeply moving to you personally, but replicating that meaning to others will never happen unless you compress the arduous complexity into beautiful simplicity. This is true of science, technology, writing a sentence, and understanding your own life.

Ideas aren't plans. Ideas can't sail the boat. Ideas are just a lighthouse.

Here's a real-life example. Parenting. It isn't easy. You have to account for every emotional climate, escalating intellectual challenges, and dangers both existential and physical. Creating a step-by-step map would be madness. Instead, my idea for parenting is helping my kids be kind, smart, and strong. Forget the details. No map. Just keep paddling the lifeboat towards those three guiding lights. This parenting tactic can scale. Thirty years from now maybe my kids will be parents. A step-by-step map of parenting in 2022 wouldn't be that helpful. Boat technology, weather, and climate will all be different, but the lighthouse will still be doing its thing. The kids can motor towards strong, smart, and kind with the same sense of adventure KT and I do today because it is a simple idea.

If you want to run any number of miles for a specific time, the guiding idea is also simple. You will have to spend time running miles. This is unavoidable. People have tried other methods. Nick Bare is a former Army Ranger and bodybuilder who decided to run a marathon. He finished well over four hours, and not until dropping weight and logging fifty plus miles/week was he able to accomplish his goal of running a sub-three-hour marathon, finishing at 2:56:27. Lance Armstrong—doping or not—was one of the greatest cyclists the world has ever seen. Even with his truly world-class aerobic conditioning, his best marathon time ever was 2:59:36. That's an amazing time, sure, but it's not even comparable to his elite cycling ability. You can lift, bike, swim, and jazzercise yourself until you're the fittest damn non-runner in the world, but if you want to be better at running, well... The point—the idea of this entire chapter—is so simple and unavoidable that you might as well shrug and re-read the title. Yeah. Looks like we're running.

That's the big idea. To get better at the thing, you must do the thing. The thing is running. More miles? Yes. More quickly? Sometimes. More slowly? Most of the time. More intentionally? Yes. All the time. You will run on purpose. Heck, what am I saying? It's week five. You're already running more intentionally.

In week five of training for the Disney Marathon, I run twenty-six miles with a long run of eleven miles. I still feel good. Wednesday of this week is the four-year anniversary of wrapping chemo and being declared cancer free. For that day's workout, I run four miles. In between the slow warm-up and cool-down, I run four rounds of 400m at a sub-seven-minute pace, and I feel like I'm flying. Time is the personal placeholder of value, and I promised myself I'd always value the time where my body gets to work. I spend time working for my body, and in return, if I'm lucky, my body works for me. This partnership between me and my body—this time together—it is a gift.

The daily details of my training plan were nothing fancy. I built the plan myself off of a few different plans I saw in Runner's World. I'm not going to give you a running plan here. You can find that anywhere. I'm simply going to give you a running idea with a few principles.

The idea: Run longer or faster.
Principle One: The long run is sacred.
Principle Two: Run fast twice a week.
Principle Three: If not running fast, run easy. Like, super chill.
Principle Four: Increase mileage no more than ten percent per week.

If God Himself can guide a chosen people with ten commandments and a philosophy—for you pagans, that philosophy is to love the Lord your God with all your heart, soul, and mind—then surely I can guide a few wannabe runners with four principles and an idea. These aren't even commandments. They're just the basics of polarized training.

Polarized training? What is that? Funny I should ask.

Polarized training is the elimination of moderate intensity. You operate at polar ends of the effort spectrum. You either work out at high intensity, or you work out at low intensity. As it relates to the idea of this chapter, you're either building endurance to run farther, or you're building speed to run faster. Oddly enough, marathon day is one of the few times you'll find yourself running at a moderate intensity.

Low Intensity? High Intensity? Who decides these intensities? Funny I should ask. Man, I just keep walking right into these layups.

You! You decide the intensity. Or, more specifically, your cardiovascular system decides the intensity. This is where that as-cool-as-James-Bond running watch comes in handy. Low intensity is quantitatively defined by workouts where your heart rate stays below seventy-seven percent of its maximum rate. You should breathe comfortably in this effort, and if you were subjectively judging the difficulty by using the same kind of one-to-ten scale that teenage boys use to rank hot chicks, this workout should feel it's somewhere between one and four. It's almost embarrassing to be seen at this pace. High intensity is defined by workouts where your heart rate stays above ninety-three percent of your max heart rate. This is a seven to ten on our teenage boy, perceived effort scale. You'll be breathing as hard as you possibly can after just a few minutes. It's extremely hard and you won't last long (that's what she said).

Okay, nice. So how does one calculate their max heart rate? Great question. It's like I'm writing in the low intensity zone. Am I embarrassed at the lack of effort in these paragraph transitions? Of course I am, but I'm also super chill. Turns out writing is super easy when you stop trying so hard. That's a great insight for someone who would like to do more writing. Now let's answer the question.

Max heart rate can be calculated in a few ways:

Option A is a supervised lab test. You've seen these in Gatorade commercials, where the athlete is running on a treadmill with the fighter pilot mask from Top Gun strapped to their face. This is a world-class athlete's version of plugging into The Matrix to realize they're a real person who gets tired. This isn't the way you're going to do it.

Option B is a field test. Before the field test, be sure to get a great warm up. Get your joints through a full range of motion with various calisthenics, then a good ten to fifteen minutes of jogging with progressive speed. You'll want to hit max speed for a few seconds more than once. Then, you do the test, which is simply to give all you have. I like the 5K for this, which is 3.1 miles. You run hard, almost tapping yourself out, and with a half mile left, you try to run so fast that you don't think you'll be able to hold on to the finish, and when you feel like you're fading, summon the power of your ancestors by yelling your last name to get every last drop of oxygenated blood. Give it all you've got. Whatever your heart rate monitor hits in the last two hundred yards, that'll be your max heart rate.

Option C is less painful. Just estimate your max heart rate. Here are the formulas I've seen:

- [220 – Age] – most common and widely used maximum heart rate formula
- [207 – 0.7 x Age] – more precise formula, adjusted for people over the age of forty
- [211 – 0.64 x Age] – slightly more precise formula, adjusted for generally active people

Max heart rate declines with age. Women typically have a max heart rate of approximately ten beats per minute higher than men. Those are just things to consider. I used the first formula and the adjusted non-forty-year-old formula, and my max estimates were 184bpm and 188bpm respectively. However, individuals vary widely. Like Ted Lasso said, "All people are different people." I haven't seen above 180bpm on my Apple Watch in the last year of regular exercise. And before you jump to any false conclusions, know that I occasionally go extremely hard. I did the three-mile field test, CrossFit WODs, Peloton PRs, and sprints, and haven't topped 180bpm. So I'm below the estimate. Probably means I'm going to die young, which is at least twenty-two percent of why I'm trying to get more fit.

Once satisfied that you know your max heart rate, you can define your intensity levels by heart rate. Mine are as follows:

- Low intensity: Stay under 139bpm (less than 77% of max HR, 180bpm)

- High Intensity: Get above 167bpm (over 93% of max HR, 180bpm)
- Moderate Intensity: Between 139-167bpm. Avoid running here.

Why all this math? You hate math. Your anti-intellectualism is predictable, but this math helps amateurs get pleasing results, like using measuring cups when you're a rookie in the kitchen.

You're going to spend dozens, potentially hundreds of hours running. If you understand yourself and tailor the effort of those runs for *you*, that time will yield the greatest reward. Rewards create anticipation. Anticipation creates repetition, and repetition is the surest path to success. I want us to keep going! If the math is *really* too much for you, I won't squabble. Just run most of your runs at a pace where you can talk full sentences without pausing for air, and then run hard twice a week. For more info, dive into the book *80/20 Running: Run Stronger and Race Faster by Training Slower* by Matt Fitzgerald. Fitzgerald is a prolific fitness writer who dives deep on this exact topic, and it's exactly what it sounds like. Do eighty percent of your running at low intensity, and twenty percent of your running at moderate or (preferably) high intensity. Here's the benefits of this polarized training, straight from the book jacket:

- Runs will become more pleasant and less draining.
- You'll carry less fatigue from one run to the next.
- Your performance will improve in the few high-intensity runs.
- Your fitness levels will reach new heights.

There you go.

Armed with your maximum heart rate and the knowledge of proper training intensity, we can discuss the principles and then the idea.

Principle One: The long run is sacred. Have you ever seen the scheduling analogy of filling up a jar? A teacher fills a glass jar with big rocks and asks the students if it's full. Some students say yes, and some say no. The teacher dumps in pebbles and shakes the jar until the pebbles fill in all the cracks. A few student "no's" turn into "yes's", but some maintain there are more cracks to fill in. The teacher then pours in sand, shaking and sifting until there is not a single space or crack of light to be seen. Now all the students say the jar is full. Nothing else could possibly fit. The teacher pulls out a bottle of water, slowly pours it on top of the jar, and the sand darkens a shade as the moisture crowds out every pocket of air in the jar. The brilliance of the analogy is about sequencing. If the teacher puts the elements into the jar in any other order—starting with the sand and saving the big rocks for last—then all the elements won't fit. When you're building your running plan, your biggest, most unwieldy rock is the long run.

The long run is not a long run. It's *the* long run. It's the longest run you will do all week, and depending on your experience, it could be the longest run of your life. For KT in her first marathon, she will run the longest run of her life five times with runs of fifteen, seventeen, nineteen, twenty, and finally 26.2 miles. She'll run fifteen miles twice, actually, but the second time it will just be the long run of the week. These runs happen at low intensity, so someone aiming for a sub-four-hour marathon will probably be training long in the 9:30-11 minute-per-mile pace. The time required makes this the most difficult run to execute. Even if you can walk right out your front door to run, you're easily into a three-hour commitment. Schedule this time first, and don't let it be interrupted.

You probably need to do long runs on a weekend. I've tried early mornings, running the eighteen miles to my office where I had a shower and a change of clothes left there the day before, but unless you wake up at 4:00 a.m. to fuel, hydrate and have a bowel moment, the super early run is an injury risk and a pain in the ass.

If you put it on the weekend, you will have all sorts of activities and holidays that threaten the effort. This is just unavoidable. My long runs are on Saturday. KT's are on Sunday. We trade off watching kids. We will be running on Thanksgiving weekend and Christmas weekend, packing our running gear into a car for her brother's and parents' houses, and onto a plane for my brother's house. It is a hassle, but if you can make the long run the immovable rock of your schedule, the rest of the training fills in easily around it.

As for the long run itself, the first week should be roughly twenty to thirty percent of the time it will take you to run your race goal. I'm training for a four-hour marathon, so my first long run is seven miles, and takes me sixty-nine (nice) minutes to complete. My average heart rate is 137bpm. I will increase my long run by about ten minutes a week, three weeks in a row. Then, on week four, I will decrease the mileage in the long run, and I will run it fast. As I wrote in the last chapter, week 4 was a deload week where my long run dropped from the nine miles of week 3 to the seven miles in week 4. I ran five of those seven miles at 7:35 minute-per-mile pace, and after the first five minutes, my heart rate stayed between 160-168bpm for the run. And now we're here in week 5, and my long run is eleven miles. I'll keep on growing it over the months until I can tackle 26.2.

Principle Two: Run fast twice a week.

There's going to be soreness. I am typically sore when I run farther than I've ever run before. Also—and I blame middle age for this—I am typically sore if I sprint or come close to sprinting. If I'm going to run far on Saturday, then that really only gives me Monday through Thursday to run fast. I like taking Thursday and Sunday off if I can, so I'm jamming in two faster runs between Monday and Wednesday. These runs are usually some form of interval, hill, or tempo run. The five fast miles of week 4 would be an example of tempo run. Finding a tough pace and holding it for an extended period of time, anywhere from twenty to sixty minutes. Interval runs are pushing yourself beyond a pace that you can hold for a long time, and jogging very slowly in between intervals to recover. My interval run of week five is a four-mile run. I jog one mile to warm up, then run a quarter-mile at a sub-seven-minute pace, followed by a quarter mile at an eleven-minute pace, and repeat that three more times. The intervals last for two miles before my fourth and final mile is jogged to cool down. Hills are hills. I have a steep hill that's about one-fifth of a mile. I run up it hard, spiking my heart rate, and then jog it back down. I usually do this eight to twelve times as the middle part of an hour-long run.

I'll add this about Principle Two. If you only run fast once a week, it's not the worst thing in the world. There's a reason these are principles, not commandments. If you're building a ton of volume, like going from ten miles a week to finishing a marathon, then you should be focused on long, easy miles. The fast running is not the priority. If you're running a shorter race, then you can commit to more frequent speed.

Principle Three: If you're not running fast, run easy. Like, super chill. You're trying to get your body to adapt, and it can't adapt if it's always beaten down. When you see someone on Instagram posting about their twelve-mile run at a "nice and easy" seven-minute-per-mile pace, that means absolutely nothing to you. They may be lying about easy. They may not know what easy means. They may be a hell of a lot faster and fitter than you are, and that really was easy. The thing is, all the science says that training speed and endurance in the same run is not giving you a double helping of fitness. So if you're not getting extra fitness, why run in a way that's harder to sustain? The vast majority of a runner's adaptation occurs at low intensity. Your joints get stronger. Your tendons stiffen. Your muscles push and catch the weight. Also, recovery occurs, and that's where gains are made at the cellular level. I don't know what the hell it actually means, but the scientific benefit of easy running is increasing mitochondrial density. Remember mitochondria? The powerhouse of the cell? Yeah, I went to high school too. Increasing the density of the cell's powerhouse has gotta be a good thing.

I'm getting out of my depth. Let's focus. The real juice of Principle Three is that you won't run yourself into the ground, physically or emotionally, and science says it makes you faster and stronger. So just get on board. Run easy.

Principle Four: Increase your mileage no more than ten percent per week. Early on, this will mostly be accounted for in your long run, but the whole week will start to look beefier over time. Ten percent isn't a hard rule, but don't mess with it too much. You need to keep increasing, but if you increase too much too quickly, you melt your wings and never fly again. Injury. It's bad. Ten percent is enough, and it won't take long before you wish it were less.

The idea: Run longer or faster. I'm done being cute. Let's hit it on the nose. Run longer **OR** faster. Bold, all-caps, and underlined, and not underlined like a hyperlink. Underlined like, "Hey, dummy, this is emphasized!" If you're running longer, don't run faster. If you're running faster, don't run longer. The dual strains of faster *and* longer aren't helpful. If you're running longer, do that. If you're running faster, do that. If you do focus on of those independently in regular rotation according to the principles, then yeah, you will eventually be able to run longer or faster. The "and" is for race day.

And on that day? Trust your body. You've showed up for it. It will show up for you.

Alright, let's wrap this chapter. Did I make that complicated enough? With what we've covered above, you can build a skeleton program for just about anyone. Running coaches would probably disagree for "professional" reasons, but it's true. Even if you're 150 pounds overweight, you can start a program. Maybe there won't be much running in the beginning, but if you focus on heart rate and time, and you start scheduling with your long run at an easily achievable length for your fitness level, then you won't overwork yourself. The speed will come when you're ready. Don't worry about the performance. Everything in the training is just training. Performance only counts on race day, and even that is just a data point of distance and speed. What would you do with that besides examine it for more training?

Run longer or faster. I don't know if it's a great idea, but it is simple.

Week 6
Run to Live: The Essence of Cross-Training

Technically, the best running I've ever seen was at the Beijing Olympics in 2008. I've never really attended any other running competition. I didn't go when my friends ran track in high school. I didn't go when my girlfriend ran cross country in college. I *did* stand on the sideline of a half marathon for ten minutes as I waited for KT to jog by. We were engaged at that point, so I'd decided to be slightly less self-absorbed. Plus, my parents were in town and I wanted to support her. I don't know; it seemed like the right thing to do. My point is, with my limited experience as a running spectator, the Beijing Olympics should *easily* be the most impressive running I've ever witnessed. It is not.

I'm going to tell a story. It's relevant, I think. But first, as its subtitle implies, this chapter is about cross-training. For real runners, cross-training can be a boring necessity. For non-runners who find ourselves running, cross-training can be a beautiful opportunity to love who we are.

The most impressive running I've ever witnessed was on the track of Blue Valley High School when I was fourteen years old. It was the summer right before my freshman year, and I was one of roughly seventy-five boys who thought they would play football for the BVHS Tigers. I haven't kept up, but I can tell you that in Kansas during the year 2000, class 6A football was a big deal. Middle schools were converging, bringing a new mix of dudes together, a new mix of hierarchy, a new mix of teenage, alpha-dog bullshit. I don't care how much I mature, deep down I'll always feel that being the toughest guy in school is a state championship of the soul. No one can ever take that away from you. I was never at the pinnacle of this toughness hierarchy, but I also wasn't at the bottom. Like the other seventy-four boys, I wanted to prove I was closer to the top than the middle. Did I care about emotional courage and loving myself for who I was? Don't make me laugh. These were the first days of weight training and conditioning for the Class of 2004, and manhood was on the line. *Everything* was on the line.

For context, I was 6'2" and 155 pounds when I was fourteen. I was a pencil neck, a dweeb, a string bean. I pretended otherwise. At that age in life, we're probably all trying on personalities, propping up our sense of belonging with a pretense when the reality is that we have no idea who we actually are. I don't want to incorporate too many notes from my personal therapy sessions, but I was consciously aware of my own pretense when I was fourteen. My older brother was *actually* the toughest kid in school, and he had *actually* won a state championship, *and* he had over a 4.0 GPA. My older brother Joe was a confident introvert with good manners, and he was the hardest worker in the room. If you're scaling for midwestern preference, he was exactly who your dad wished you were. That last part is probably not true (I have a great dad), but that's the sense my adolescent mind had cobbled together. I'd been homeschooled up to that point, and social interaction was scary. I wanted to be liked. I knew I wasn't my brother, but the way I believed other people saw him was almost exactly how I wanted them to see me. This projection of wishful identity is a strong element for anyone's choice of hero, but I had evidence that the gap between him and me was real. He would be a senior that year, and the varsity guys were finishing their workouts when us freshman arrived. We walked into the weight room, and there he was. 6'1" and 240 pounds, built exactly like a college linebacker. He was doing power cleans, a lift for which he would temporarily hold the school record of 325 pounds if memory serves. The other freshmen watched him, dripping with sweat yet totally comfortable moving weight none of us could move.

One of the other freshmen—we'll give him the fake name Jerry—Jerry turned to me and asked, "That's your brother?"

I beamed with pride and said, "Yeah."

Then Jerry said the worst thing he could say. He said the thing that I believed everyone thought but never said. Jerry said, "What happened to *you*."

And that's how he said it. Not with an emphasis on "happened" or a question mark at the end. He emphasized "you" and put a period on it. Case closed. His mind was made up. It was a devastating moment. I was devastated.

Don't cry for me, Argentina. I'm good. I made it. I won a football state championship my senior year, and I graduated with over a 4.0 GPA, and, as I grew up, I discovered enough of me that was like my brother to also be grateful that I was not exactly him. I was never even close to being the toughest kid in school, but moments like the one with Jerry initiated my own form of resiliency. In fact, I tapped into some resiliency mere minutes after Jerry's insult.

The coaches corralled all the freshmen to the track and broke us up into groups. This was a fitness evaluation, and we were going to run a mile. Kids my age in eastern Kansas ran a mile as often as they went to the beach. Inexperience allowed me to believe that running fast was simply about overcoming my own pain tolerance, and, given the events of the morning, I was ready to prove how tough I was. I ended up near the front of my pack, and on that last lap, when my lungs were bursting and my legs were filled with acid, I didn't relent. I finished in the top five of my group with a young PR, roughly 6:15. The guys who beat me didn't smoke me. I think the top guy finished around six minutes. I was right near the top.

Then the next group ran.

BeeJay McLoyd was the best athlete in our class. He could go from standing to full-speed in an instant, and made cuts with no latency. He'd be a starting varsity receiver as a freshman that year. Normally a class-clown type, BeeJay now stood silent and poised at the starting line. I think BeeJay knew that he was different than most of us, that he had real potential to take football far, and he wanted to prove that difference on day one. The whistle blew, and the group started running, and it wasn't more than half a lap before the front group was less than five guys. By the end of the first lap, there were only three, and by the half mile mark, the front group was only BeeJay and a second string running back named Bryce Benton.

This was the most impressive running performance I've ever seen. I knew Bryce was a real runner. He had won a lot of meets in middle school. But I'd never watched it. BeeJay was a sprinter, but he had run with Bryce in track practice. BeeJay knew that he had never run the mile nearly as fast as Bryce, but like me, BeeJay thought that maybe it was about tolerance. He gave it everything he had, and for the first time ever, I watched the best athlete I'd ever met give it everything and have it not be enough. BeeJay finished his mile something like 5:10. He was about to topple over, and he said, "I didn't know I could do that." Those are PR words, and it was impressive, but it wasn't anywhere close to Bryce Benton's 4:50. The crazy part? By the time BeeJay came across the line looking like he'd keel over, Bryce was looking mostly recovered.

Our head coach was something of a local legend, and when he gathered all of us around he said, "I will never forget the name Bryce Benton after what I saw today." Well, Coach, me neither. Twenty-two years later and the memory is clear. My friends who were there that day still remember too. The parameters of Benton's excellence were narrow, but that's what a personal experience is. I have no idea if Bryce shared all my insecurities about how he wished others saw him, but in the eyes of a few of us, he shined as one of the toughest guys we'd ever seen. So for us, he is immortal.

In week six of training for the Disney Marathon, I run twenty-eight miles with a long run of twelve miles. I finish the audiobook of *Running to the Edge: A Band of Misfits and the Guru Who Unlocked the Secrets of Speed*, and I begin the audiobook *Running with Sherman: The Donkey with the Heart of a Hero*. They have me thinking about the social impacts of running and wondering if the biggest mistake of my training regimen is how isolated I am in my efforts. I run my twelve miles on Saturday at an 8:54/mi pace with an average heart rate of 140bpm. I'm hurting a bit at the end, and regret peaking over my easy pace on multiple occasions. It'll be fine, right?

I did four days of cross-training this week that consisted of the following:

- Thirty minutes of Peloton yoga
- Squats, pull-ups, push-ups, core, and twenty minutes on the Concept2 Rower
- Deadlifts, shoulder press, core
- Rec league basketball

The argument Capital-R runners make for cross-training is that it balances your muscles, enhances mobility, aids running economy, and lowers the chance of injury. I love those benefits. Who wouldn't? If you're focused purely on running, just throw in twenty to thirty minutes of something different three times a week and you're good. Variation is relief. I don't think I'm being too dismissive about that either. I know some incredible runners, and their cross-training is not very complex. But if you're a little-R runner, I'd like to suggest that cross-training is something else that's more valuable than an aid or a balance or an enhancement. Cross-training is your opportunity to see yourself more clearly.

What's the point of the long story above? Since this book is for runners, the point of the story is a chiasmus: you either live to run, or you run to live. The story is about teenage boys, and only Bryce was a runner. The rest of us boys—in our minds—were football players. The average length of a football play is four seconds. How fast you run a mile may matter less than your taste in music. In a group of seventy-four football players, running the mile wasn't the training. Running the mile was something separate that enhanced the experience. I have entire months of near-collapse football workouts and grueling practices that I cannot remember. That's probably good. There's an aspect of routine that is necessarily unmemorable to allow you to grind through years of hard work and improvement. That mile, though? Its prime benefit was that it was *not* the training. It was something else, and because it was unique, it can be cherished in its own way. Over two decades later, I still suspect the seed of my interest in running is the combination of defending Jerry's insult with a one-mile PR before witnessing Bryce and BeeJay's duel. I experienced in that moment something I would intellectualize after reading a quote I've already shared: "One run can change your day. Many runs can change your life."

That running changes your life is spiritually true, but it's also factually true. As your physical condition improves, activities that were taxing become simply fun. With that in mind, the following is the most helpful advice I can give you about cross-training: make your cross-training about you. You may be tempted to make the cross-training about running, but running makes you a better runner, not cross-training. So go rock-climbing or skiing or skateboarding. Play flag football or kickball or ultimate frisbee. What do you love to do? Or what did you love doing when you were younger that you haven't done in a while? You're building all this fitness. Use it to get some life.

I find life in rec league basketball. As important as football was to me, the athletic love of my life has always been basketball. The first time I recognized symptoms of the cancer growing in my body was playing a morning pickup game. Five minutes of playing felt like an entire day, so I left, and I didn't stop breathing hard for another hour. After chemo, I got caught up in rehabbing my entire life, and only a year ago did I get back to playing ball, and I can't overstate this: Basketball is maybe the most fun I'm capable of having at this stage of life. Basketball is nostalgia. It's the athletic version of reuniting with dear friends you only get to see once or twice a year. Basketball is clarity. I'm so immersed in the present intensity of competition that none of life's stress can fuzzy the experience. Basketball is balance. When I come home after a game, I'm energized and eager to give time to my family because I've satisfied my desire for me-time so completely. Basketball is the thing I do to help me love everything else I do. In short, basketball is my perfect cross-training from running, and thanks to the running, I'm playing better than I have since my early twenties. It's much easier to play well when you're not gassed in the first five minutes.

If running sticks for you, if it becomes your primary source of fitness, then you will understand it is only cross-training for life. You will eventually find a capacity for action far greater than you've experienced in your non-running life. I hope it comes as a comfort to you—as it has for me—that this capacity is not a sacrifice. The running is an aid, an enhancement. The running balances your life and decreases the chance that you become injured and unable to live as you wish.

Week 7
Food Is Fuel

I felt smart once. It was one of my first classes in college, a communications course. The professor presented the class with a factoid. In a study, drinkers of Mountain Dew were especially likely to experience tooth decay prior to middle age (don't hassle me for specifics, this was eighteen years ago). The question we college students were asked to consider in a collegiate way was this: *Why?* They love hitting you with the big questions in college, don't they? A couple of students posited straightforward answers like sugar and flavor. *Psh, what K-12 thinking.* The teacher—excuse me, professor—didn't say they were wrong, exactly, but he did keep fielding answers, so I weighed in.

"I mean, Mountain Dew is probably not great for your teeth, but, it's like, people who drink Mountain Dew probably aren't taking great care of themselves. Maybe people who drink Mountain Dew are also the same people who don't brush their teeth."

The professor pretended not to be impressed, but we both knew. He segued my insight to a socioeconomic study about Mountain Dew sales per capita, and the highest rates occurred in regions where people were more likely to live in poverty and had less access to quality dental care. The poor and under-resourced most often Do the Dew because it's cheap, distributed everywhere and never goes bad. The lesson was to not mistake correlation with causation. Tooth decay is a poverty issue, not a Mountain Dew issue.

That's basically what I said, right? These Mountain Dew drinkers are a type. Boom! Me: a genius at eighteen. Maybe not a boy genius, and not quite a man-genius either, but definitely a—okay, no. Not a genius. Still, I was on the cusp of understanding something about misinformation and my health.

This chapter is about nutrition and hydration, and I don't know why, but people love telling you what you should and shouldn't put in your body. It's one of the weirdest, most persistent annoyances about human beings. When it comes to explaining to others what is good and bad about food, drinks, and drugs, Americans get pathological in ways only rivaled by sex and religion. I hate when people are extremely defensive about their non-existent diet plan (see addicts, gluttons, or sloths). I hate when people are extremely offensive about their specific diet plan (see vegans, carnivores, and dickheads). This chapter will throw away all that bullshit so you can think about food exactly the same way I do.

Just kidding. We'll do it like the other chapters. I'll say some stuff and then you can think whatever you think while I remain blissfully unaware of whether or not I've been a good, bad, or neutral influence in your life. Set it and forget it. That's my style. I'm the Ronco Showtime Rotisserie of writers. Put that last sentence on my tombstone.

In week seven of training for the Disney Marathon, I'm going to run thirty-one miles with a long run of thirteen miles. The great debate is whether I should just extend that long run into 13.1 miles and call it a half marathon? I mean, whatever man. I'm not going to do it. Whether I'm talking about training runs, fashion, or sex, my mentality is, "Nothing to prove." I'm not running that extra point-one. I'm not going to worry about anything off-plan until I run the City of Oaks half marathon in five weeks. I'm gonna run for a half PR in that race no matter what my training would otherwise suggest. Until then, I run the miles, stay hydrated, and eat lots of food.

Yes, back to food.

It is difficult to sort through all the literature, recommendations, and anecdotes to decide what is and isn't good for us to consume. When we make a choice about what we will eat, we tend to cling to that choice long after we've seen evidence to the contrary. Mountain Dew is a fine example. It's terrible for you, right? Well, I'm not so sure. Ultramarathoner Zach Bitter set a world record in the one hundred-mile ultra with a time of eleven hours and nineteen minutes. His average pace is a sub-three-hour marathon. That's a 6:48 mile for one hundred miles! Naturally, that got attention, and Zach went on the Joe Rogan Experience. Amongst other things, he said, "I did a 100K(kilometer) race, and I did nothing but Mountain Dew." Let me add that Zach and Joe talk for ninety minutes, and they say the word "diet" over twenty times. Mountain Dew is not the only item on Zach Bitter's grocery list. Still, I Googled the hell out of Mountain Dew and running research. Know what's special about it? Not a damn thing. It's not "bad" or "good" or anything definitive. It's just liquid sugar, basically a Powerade with some caffeine. An hour of research on the fifth most popular soft drink by revenue in America only reinforced something I already knew: what your body needs to consume is highly dependent on what your body is attempting to do.

As a group of people whose bodies are attempting to run farther, there are some basic principles about food. The most important principle is...

Actually, before I get into the rule, let me issue a warning about the scale and the mirror. Some of us may see skinny runners and think that skinny is beautiful. It's subjective of course. I have too much macho baggage to envy the skin-and-bone aesthetic, but I understand the draw of change. When you begin to see cheekbones and a jawline emerge from the cheeks-that-beer-built, you might as well be Daniel Craig emerging from the ocean in *Casino Royale*. Get me some super tiny shorts! That's all great stuff. Seeing those results in the mirror is wonderful. However, don't let yourself be consumed. The scale stops going down at some point. How will you feel when it goes up? If you have any emotions tied to your weight, don't step on a scale. It's just a number, and there's no specific amount of gravity's pull on your mass that will satisfy you. I have a rack that holds all my running medals. On it is a quote from Jordan Peterson that says, "What you aim at determines what you see." Aim higher than the scale beneath your feet.

Okay, rule number one is:

Food is fuel. I'm not getting into dietary specifics. My favorite book on dietary behavior is Michael Pollan's *In Defense of Food*. The entire book can be boiled down to a sentence: Eat real food, not too much, mostly plants. It's an excellent principle, but marathon training is one of the few times I venture happily from the principle. Why? I want more fuel.

Know this about me. I'm from the Midwest. I've looked at a scale and seen 270 pounds. I know what it means to eat a lot of food. I've also lost weight. Prior to this marathon training, I weighed 210 pounds and was tracking everything I ate on My Fitness Pal. When I started the training block, I stopped tracking. I'm doing my best to eat real food, but I'm also, occasionally, eating with reckless abandon. *I've got a long run tomorrow*, is my Friday night mantra as I inject eight slices of pizza into my veins. And guess what? My weight has not fluctuated at all. I was doing intermittent fasting before this training block. Now, I eat breakfast every day. I've added an extra meal to my diet, no weight gain. Routinely, I'm eating dinner and then eating more dinner. I believe the term is "having seconds." The scale doesn't blink. I check to see if the scale is broken. The scale isn't broken. The guiltless eating is the upside of running really long distances. With little exercise, my caloric needs to hold weight are about 2,400 a day. A nine-mile run burns another 1,300 calories. That's a lot of extra food. Thirteen hundred calories is three Quarter Pounders from McDuck's! If you start running faster or longer, you probably need to change your diet, and it's a high likelihood that means eating more, not less.

This update on my static body weight isn't justification to eat junk food, even if I will turn on Sheryl Crow's "My Favorite Mistake" as I'm stirring a brownie mix together. This update is to enforce rule number one, that food is fuel. Your body is a machine ruled by physical law and biological limitations. There is a lot of truth that being lighter means being faster. That's advice for a lifetime of running, not a single training block. There is some research about fasted running expediting physical adaptations, but my scientific opinion is that's malarkey. There's far more research indicating that better fuel is more beneficial than an empty gas tank. Eventually, if you run for enough years, if you're curious and experimental, you'll find what works for you. I'm writing this for us amateurs: We shouldn't limit caloric resources during a training block. We need our fuel.

The good news is that a lot of that fuel should be carbs. I love carbs. Carbs are the most efficient source of energy. In fact, as you're increasing your weekly mileage by fifteen plus miles per week over the course of this training block, a carb shortage is painful and unwise. Running on low fuel increases injury risk. Our worst running happens when we're tired and depleted. Our form breaks down and we make bad pacing decisions. Then we're tired and sore the next day and mistakes compound.

Running on low fuel can also turn runs into a sufferfest. Remember, we want eighty percent of our running to be easy, and if we're under-fueled, we can run slow and it still won't be easy. The biggest benefit of easy running is that it encourages continuous running. This isn't just true of a single run or a few months of training, but it's true as a lifestyle. If you really want to be fit—and I use that term for shape *and* functionality—then creating lifelong habits is your best bet. The easiest way to do that is to avoid doing something that makes running more painful, like starving yourself of your best energy source: carbs.

Not making life painful is my best reason to eat plenty of fuel. If you only run this one marathon, your body will revert back to whatever it was before you were running. No need to starve yourself for a yo-yo experience. And what if you don't revert back? What if you end up making running a long-term part of your life? Well, how many truly overweight people do you see running twenty-five miles a week? No need to make an enemy of food in that situation. You will need your fuel. With either approach, might as well eat.

Three quick hitters:

When you eat matters. I like carbs an hour before running, but do what's comfortable for your run. Replenishment is more vital. You need carbs and protein within ninety minutes of finishing your workout to give yourself the best chance of recovering and strengthening for future runs. The standard is a ratio of 4g of carbs to 1g of protein. Don't overthink it though. Your body is incredibly smart at using what you give it. Just try to give it some quality carbs and protein. I use smoothies and protein shakes a lot since I'm rarely in the mood to house broccoli and salmon right after a twelve-mile run.

Add electrolytes. Sodium is the most important. Whether it's salting your water or buying an electrolyte mix with a fuller profile, electrolytes will greatly help with cramps and fatigue. My heart rate drops significantly on runs where I've added electrolyte mixes to my preparation. Electrolytes are essential elements my muscles need to fire, so if I have a higher volume of electrolytes in my blood, my heart doesn't have to pump as hard to send the resources. It's like overstuffing a suitcase so you don't have to pay for a second bag. How much electrolytes you'll need will depend on how you feel, so start experimenting with different amounts so you're comfortable by race day. My favorite supplement options are LMNT drink mix and BPN Electrolytes.

Know about glycogen. Glycogen depletion is a key limiting factor in races that last more than two hours. Glycogen is the most efficient form of fuel that your body can store, and most people don't store enough for more than ninety-minutes' worth of running. Depleting this fuel source is what happens to runners who talk about "hitting the wall" or "bonking." Some research suggests that your autonomic brain fights your conscious mind when you're running low on glycogen, slowing you down so that you won't run the fuel gauge down to E. I like this mental image of a gas gauge. The harder you run, the more quickly you burn the gas. Meaning, if you're concerned with running performance, glycogen should be topped off as often as possible. This means eating carbs while running. The gold standard for multi-hour runs is eating 60g of carbs per hour. Limiting factor is going to be what your stomach can handle while running, so do some gastric experimentation with different carb sources on long runs. You want to have a reliable source by the time you get to race day. We'll talk about this more as we get closer to race day, but for runs over an hour, I like having an energy gel or a sports drink about midway through. For three hour runs, I'll continuously be taking in gels and drinks to prevent my body from recognizing glycogen depletion. There are beans, chews, and all sorts of other options formulated for runners. Try them all. If you find what works for you, you'll be glad you did.

Week 8
Sleep and Recovery

"They"—heavy scare quotes—say a person loses one hour of sleep per night in their first year as a parent. Stack those 365 hours together and that's fifteen days lost sleep. Can you imagine such exhaustion? I don't have to. That deficit is my reality. Walter is two years old. Winnie is seven months old. KT and I love our kids more than sleep. Barely. And we control what we can control. No alcohol, no nicotine, no medications, relax before bed, avoid blue light, blackout curtains, cool room, and barring a Kansas City Chiefs late game, I'm always in bed before 10:00 p.m. In fact, KT and I usually take two nights to watch a single movie because of our early bed time. In a perfect world, neither of us would be waking up for early morning baby-feedings, but compromise is love and love is compromise. As the stoic Seneca said, "I pay the taxes of life gladly." The broccoli will never taste like Ben & Jerry's. The Ben & Jerry's will never be healthy. I eat both foods gladly.

But this chapter isn't about food. It's about sleep and recovery.

Hopefully you've lived enough life to have some personal experience with the benefits of sleep. If you're a "sleep when I'm dead" type, well, you're not wrong, but for running, the guidance is simple. The more you run, the more you'll need sleep. Sleep isn't just about physical recovery and energy replenishment. Sleep is also the time your brain reinforces new skill sets. Studies show a thirty percent improvement in newly learned motor skills after a full night's sleep. Conversely, sleep deprivation is linked to a rapid increase in chance of injury. Have you ever rolled your ankle? Was the error truly random or a breakdown in motor skill? Research suggests physical misjudgments skyrocket in a sleep-deprived brain. And do you ever have gut problems, or as I less elegantly call them: the mid-run shits? A lack of sleep increases cortisol (aka the stress hormone) which increases gastrointestinal problems. Where are you with vanity and performance? At caloric deficit (which happens to runners) less sleep is correlated to losing muscle and storing fat, the exact opposite of what a runner wants.

I'm not going to preach. It's the twenty-first century. Everyone knows sleep is a kingmaker. If you want to have your mind blown about how pivotal sleep is to intelligence, physical and emotional health, and living significantly longer, you should listen to Dr. Matthew Walker on any number of podcasts (like Joe Rogan or Tim Ferriss) or, better yet, buy his book, *Why We Sleep: Unlocking the Power of Sleep and Dreams*. This is one of my favorite recommendations, and it's legitimately life-changing knowledge.

In week 8 of training for the Disney Marathon, I should be running thirty-four miles. Instead, I'll run twelve. In last week's basketball game, a player's kneecap slammed against the outside of my knee. I finished the game despite feeling a little off. But by the time my car reached home, I could barely bend the knee. I'm in an orthopaedist's office eighteen hours later. The doctor puts me through some movements, prods the joint, and sends me to x-rays. Then I wait. And catastrophize. My little brother blew out his knee in high school football. One of my basketball teammates tore his ACL twice in three years, obliterating his college basketball experience. If the news is bad, it's not just the end of my marathon training. It's the beginning of a long and painful rehabilitation. The doc comes in and shrugs. He thinks I'm okay. It's not exactly the unshakeable scientific fact I'm hoping for, but any port in a storm. They can't see any structural damage. Most likely some deep bruising. It could take three or four weeks to feel right again, and while running won't necessarily do more damage, he thinks I should take it easy from high-impact movements to help speed the recovery.

I wrote before that injury is the worst possible outcome of training. I've thought about that, and it's not true. Death is worse than injury. Death is the worst possible outcome, and I just want that on the record so no one thinks I'm being overly dramatic. Like a lifetime prison-sentence, injury is second fiddle to death.

I read a lot of kids books to Walter, and my personal favorite by far is *Oh, the Places You'll Go!* by Dr. Seuss. It's a legitimate masterpiece. Despite being the last book published during Dr. Seuss's lifetime—he'd die of cancer a year later at the age of eighty-seven—this book is written in the future tense. The main character is a boy referred to only as "you," and he faces the journey of life. So many books try to say it all, but I'll be damned if this one doesn't pull it off. It covers the highs and lows, the confidence and fear, societal pressure, routine stagnation, isolation, resiliency, accountability, and balance. With my son on the lap of my bruised knee, I read this:

> *I'm sorry to say so*
> *but, sadly, it's true*
> *that Bang-ups*
> *and Hang-ups*
> *can happen to you.*

I've spent hundreds of hours in Alcoholics Anonymous, group therapy, and personal reflection, all spent wrestling with the process of recovery. Whether it's cancer, addiction, or a physical injury, the first step is always admitting you have a problem. You have to declare reality. That's why addict and comedian Russell Brand turns the first step of recovery into a question. "Step one: Are you a bit fucked up?" Sadly, a vast number of people stop going anywhere in life because they are unwilling to look at the thing that is hurting them and admit that it is hurting them. I haven't beaten addiction or cancer any more than I've become impervious to injury, but I am proud to have said, "Yeah, I am a bit fucked up." The hang-ups and bang-ups did happen to me, and I'm proud that I stopped lying about what they were. They were—and sometimes still are—the things that hurt me. I embraced them. And I'll be damned if I'm ever letting go. They get on top of me now and then, but that's how wrestling works. Recognize your position, and focus like hell to regain control, but don't let go. These lessons apply to your training every bit as much as they apply to life.

So I'm a bit fucked up. Fine. It's time to walk the walk, and I mean that literally because running isn't happening. I write out my week's training plan. In each running slot Monday to Saturday, I write, "Do your best." For Sunday, I write, "Rest." In the cross-training slots of each day, I write a reminder.

M - "Run YOUR race."

T - "Excellence > Winning."

W - "Success = Peace of Mind."

R - "Progress > Perfection."

F - "Recovery = Progress."

S - "Run some real miles?"

For Sunday, I write the ultimate reminder to myself, and it's only one word: "Grace."

Putting yourself back together again is accepting that you're broken. If it's not broke, you won't fix it. Still, there are degrees of acceptance. I'm still moving. I ride the Peloton for ninety-minute aerobic sessions. I spend an hour in a pool walk-jogging laps in the water. One day, I walk four miles. Another day, I jog two miles. Mostly, I let myself experience grace.

Maybe you thought we were going to talk about physical recovery in this chapter. Well, these next few sentences are it.

Drinking lots of water, eating enough food, keeping your easy runs truly easy, and getting plenty of good sleep are your best bets for physical recovery. Sure, we could have a discussion about foam rolling, ice baths, sauna, body work, cryotherapy, hyperbaric chambers, cupping, customized IV drips, or whatever you have the time and money to apply, but these additional treatments are salt on a steak. No matter how much you use, you can't turn a bottom round into a ribeye (for you non-steak folks, take my word, bottom round is tougher than Rocky Balboa and bland as Tom Bodett... Aside: can you imagine Tom Bodett yelling "Adrian"? I cannot).

Back to the point.

Emotional recovery is the most important recovery. Remember, the goal is success, and if you can't currently run a 5:30 mile for 26.2 consecutive miles, I feel confident saying you will not win your marathon. How can we be happy in the face of persistent discomfort, a never-ending escalation of work, and setbacks in scheduling, weather, injury, and performance? Well, maybe it is treating yourself to a customized IV. Maybe it's letting yourself eat Ben & Jerry's instead of broccoli. Maybe it's taking a day off. The miles will still be there tomorrow. In any case, the key is one word: grace. Have you ever heard about someone losing with grace? Or winning with grace? What does that mean? In the moments of victory and defeat, we allot status and justified pride to the winner, and we allot disappointment and shame to the loser. The gracious winner quickly eschews pride, redistributing responsibility and status to people not directly in the spotlight. The gracious loser has a tougher challenge. They must own their responsibility for the loss with confidence. Was their effort poor? They must say so. Did something pivotal happen via bad luck? They have to let go of that and focus on what they can control. But the grace doesn't happen without confidence. The confidence—sometimes as much of a show as an emotional reality—the confidence is the difference between suffering a setback and being defeated. Suffering a setback is saying, "A bad thing happened." Being defeated is saying, "I am the bad thing." A gracious loser has a bad run on a tough day. Without grace, the person is just a bad runner. The graceless mindset weakens you. Grace is strength. Grace is the dam that prevents guilt from becoming shame. We all will feel guilt in the pursuit of success. We stumble. We slump. Dr. Seuss writes:

And when you're in a Slump,
you're not in for much fun.
Un-slumping yourself
is not easily done.

You must not allow yourself to feel shame. The race is long, and you cannot give your best if you do not believe your best is yet to come. If you're having trouble believing that, remember that the best indicator of what you *truly* believe is action. Go for a run. If you can't run, walk. If you can't walk, be still, but don't give up. The action is to keep on going.

On and on you will hike,
And I know you'll hike far
and face up to your problems
whatever they are.

It's only week 8. There's plenty of time left. Rest. Work on what's broken. Keep going. Recover.

And will you succeed?
Yes! You will, indeed!
(98 and 3/4 percent guaranteed.)
KID, YOU'LL MOVE MOUNTAINS!

Hell yeah, Dr. Seuss. I'm going to rehab this knee injury. I'm going to get back on the road. I'm going to run the Disney Marathon in under four hours. And I'm going to start right now by icing my knee and watching half of a movie before going to bed at 9:00 p.m.

Week 9
The Halftime Break

The two sports that most shaped my life were basketball and football. My formative years saw most of the world through a lens of team sports, and I often call that lens back into place when I want to see something familiar in an otherwise new experience.

There are a lot of pauses in football and basketball: time-outs, quarter's end, dead time between plays. However, the halftime break is unique. Players retreat from the field of play to re-assess their approach to the game and tend to anything that needs tending. Coaches get to give a big speech if they're so inclined, get everyone fired up like they've got that blue face paint on in *Braveheart*. On average, halftime fails about half of the time. Dead hearts, hazy eyes, can't win. But sometimes, a team looks inward at just the right angle, and that new perspective changes everything.

For a twenty-week training block, week 9 is great for a halftime break. Since you'll want to spend two or three weeks tapering, this is the true halfway point of the build. This isn't a team sport, but let's pause. Let's high-five ourselves. Look at us! Who would've thought? The second half of the build will bring the seventeen to twenty-two-mile-long runs that really test our resolve. Maybe you've been lackluster, and you need an extra kick in the butt. Maybe you've had injuries and frustrations and need to take an emotional step back, find some perspective. Done correctly, the intentional pause of a halftime break can fortify you and relax you at the same time.

My halftime break is an event that KT and I designed. It's called

Row24. A group of friends and I keep a Concept 2 rowing machine running for twenty-four consecutive hours in dedication to the fight against blood cancers. Every twenty-four hours, four hundred eighty Americans are diagnosed with a blood cancer. A third of those victims will not survive. We keep the rower running, get the word out, and raise funds that the Leukemia and Lymphoma Society use to aid cancer victims and cancer research. We launched Row24 in 2019 at CrossFit Sua Sponte in Raleigh, raising almost fourteen thousand dollars in our first year. We skipped 2020 due to the coronavirus pandemic, and in 2021, we did a scaled-down version of Row24 in the backyard of our home. Despite vaccinations and increased knowledge about how to de-risk Covid-19, smaller numbers and an outside environment helped provide safety.

In week seven of training for the Disney Marathon, I'm going to run twenty-five miles with my long run replaced by Row24. I remember laying in the ICU, wires and needles hanging off of me. They woke me up every hour to draw blood. There was a constant ache in my back and hips. Rolling over left me panting with exhaustion. One of the most out-of-body experiences of my life was seeing the eight feet between my hospital bed and the toilet as utterly impossible. Minutes later, in the commercials of a Kansas Jayhawks basketball game, Eddie Bauer made their pitch. The people were hiking through the woods, balancing on moss-covered logs, and standing heroically at the edge of some scenic, wilderness overlook. It wasn't remotely cheesy. It was glorious. And I told myself that if I got healthy again, I'd never take my body for granted.

Row24 takes me back to that moment of clarity. It reminds me that the body is a blessing. This year, Row24 lends some of that perspective to marathon training. This year the event lands on a de-load week, where the long run would've been. I'm planning on rowing about four hours over the course of the day, so it's not a break from movement, but rowing is a low-impact gift of variation. Running tends to be a lot of lonely miles, but besides the midnight-to-5:00 a.m. shifts, Row24 is basically an all-day, backyard barbecue with non-stop food and friends. Big picture, Row24 is a break from myopia.

My experience of marathon training is that it takes on an outsized importance in your life. I find myself randomly telling people about my running when they ask about my plans for the weekend or what my week looks like. When a run is exceptional, I float. When a run sucks, I fret. If something comes up and I can't get my run in, well, the world has conspired to leave me in ruin. If you're the type of person who locks in, this myopia is likely. If you're extremely self-involved—which is its own kind of locked in—then you're like me, and this myopia is a certainty.

Row24 pulls me outside of myself, which is a nice way to say it pulls my head out of my ass. It forces me to think of the cancer. Confucius said, "Every man has two lives, and the second starts when he realizes he has just one." My second life didn't come until later, but the cancer diagnosis was the beginning of the end of my first life. A realization isn't always sudden, but if it's significant enough, you should create some sort of marker. Row24 is both a milestone and a tombstone. I hope for everyone who participates in the event, it's a milestone reminding them of how far we've come in the fight against cancers. For me, I hope I always see it as a tombstone, remembering the man I was so that I can be grateful for the man I am.

Is this all a bit melodramatic? Am I being even more myopic? Apologies.

The point is that the running isn't that important. Every day hundreds of people are getting the kind of news that will kill them or change them forever, and in light of humanity's true severities, a running goal becomes less stressful. No matter how a run goes, you can run it with a grateful heart simply because it is running and you're doing it.

Sometimes, a subtle shift from ambition to gratitude is exactly the right fuel for the back half of a training block.

For anyone feeling like their training has been lazy and inconsistent for the first nine weeks, perhaps it's time to revisit the message of chapter zero. Not everyone wants to run a marathon, but everyone *wants*. Do you want to know what you're *really* made of? If you want to learn about yourself, you have to re-commit. Lazy training will still let you finish the marathon. You'll get the shirt and the sticker for your car. But in your heart of hearts, you won't *be* a finisher. For the whole of training, you experienced the consistent buckling of your will. You ran less than the plan. You said you were going running but then just drove around, maybe got some food. You posted a weekly mileage on social media that was more than you actually did. There was a totality of work to be done, and you didn't finish it. If this type of thing is happening, then you're on your way to running 26.2 miles for reasons you are unaware of. All this work is gaining you so very little. That is not good. It's also okay. We're not curing cancer here. It's just running. If someone you knew had lackluster training in the first nine weeks —maybe too much cross-training, too few electrolytes, a knee injury —would you be super mean and call him a lazy bitch, or would you encourage him? Either way, this is a good time for self-evaluation. Talk to someone. Own your mistakes. Structure some form of accountability, even if that's just telling on yourself when you've had a bad run or skipped a run. The truth really does set you free.

[Extremely *Braveheart* voice]: And what will you do with that freedom? Will you fight?

[Extremely anonymous-Scottish-soldier voice]: No, of course not. We will run, and we will live.

[Still *Braveheart* voice]: Aye. And dying in our beds, many years from now, we will worry a little bit less about trading all the days from this day to that, because we never bullshitted ourselves.

It's just running. If it's causing you to lie to yourself or others, or if it's making you miserable, then maybe this week-nine halftime break is the time where you decide to drop it. That knee injury is worse than you thought. Call it quits. Then again, you know more than you used to know. You've run more than you had ever run before. Maybe it's time to realize you only have one training block for this marathon, so your second training block begins today.

Row24 is excellent. My coworkers at Cisco Systems get behind it. A local community from 12th State CrossFit gets behind it. In twenty-four hours, we row over 285,000 meters (177 miles). We laugh, watch college football, eat a ton of food, and most importantly, we annihilate our prior fundraising effort by sending over $42,000 to the Leukemia & Lymphoma Society. That money will help people. Those people will never know our little group of cancer fighters. That's okay. Society is built on the kindness of strangers, and none of us are looking for anything more. I'm spitballing slogans for 2023, and there's one I'm starting to like. It reminds me of a little bit of running. "Row24: The effort is the reward."

Week 10
Racing Versus Running: What Makes This Not Boring?

Anchorman: The Legend of Ron Burgundy is one of the best comedies of my lifetime. It's ridiculous and perfect. The movie is set in 1970's San Diego, a time before cable, when the local anchorman reigned supreme. In one scene, the close-knit news team is trying to reschedule their team pancake breakfast, and Ron Burgundy, played by Will Ferrell, has to bow out.

"Oop... I almost forgot. I won't be able to make it, fellas. Veronica and I are trying this new fad called, uh, jogging. I believe it's 'jogging' or 'yogging.' it might be a soft 'J'. I'm not sure but apparently you just run for an extended period of time! It's supposed to be wild."

Curious: Do you, my dear reader, like it when I lord my narrative power in a condescending way? I hope so, because I'm going to explain this joke to you. See, it's funny because it's anachronistic. Jogging wasn't a super common activity in the seventies. Get it? Old-timey people didn't know shit. Burgundy's not even sure how to pronounce the "j" in "jogging." But then there's also this zinger. Quote: "It's supposed to be wild." The seventies was a time when people trusted cocaine more than condoms, and they thought jogging was wild? Ha! How silly. But wait. Why does that work? This movie was released in 2004, and it assumes that its audience will know what Ron doesn't: Nothing could be more insanely boring than just running for an extended period of time. The entire joke hinges on a single premise: Running is not wild.

You're welcome, dear reader, by the way. Next time you watch

Anchorman, pause this part and explain the funny to those around you. Pay it forward. They'll be super happy you did.

What of that premise, though? Is running not wild? Is running, in fact, boring? This is a fairly common complaint from new runners building mileage. Running easy for twelve miles is a big chunk of time. The runs last as long as a movie. That's where our training is now. Will you get bored doing two hours of the same, repetitive motion? Maybe. Boredom is a personal experience. Some people will crave the two-hour break from work, news, social media, or the soul-vacuum responsibility of loving and raising their kids. Other people hate the feeling of their brain adrift. I suspect that natural discomfort is magnified by our anti-meditative, hyper-connected culture. Be forewarned: it doesn't matter what songs, podcast, or audiobook you put in your headphones; if run by yourself for hours at a time, your brain will have moments of severe, untethered drift.

In week 10 of training for the Disney Marathon, I run thirty-two miles with a long run of 13.1 miles. Not thirteen miles. I'm running the whole half, if that makes sense. My long run is on Saturday, about nineteen days since I hurt my knee. I'm ninety-nine percent sure it wasn't something worse than a bone bruise, and I've decided I'm going to really *go for it* on this long run. The Sir Walter Running Club puts on several races over the year, including the Raleigh Half. They're offering a preview run of the course on the same day as my long run. Such serendipity demands I break plan and run an extra 0.1 miles.

Dear reader, I must condescend once more: When you've been running a while, *as I have*, you'll be confident in making these types of aggressive adaptations in your own plan.

I show up to the preview run with about twenty-five other folks. I only know one guy here, but I can just tell by looking around that I'm in the bottom ten percent of performance. Their shorts are short.

Their legs are somehow stick thin and bulging with muscles at the same time. Their shoulders are skeletal and square, nothing but ball-and-joint in perfect posture. These people are faster than me.

The one guy I know is Sandy Roberts, a co-founder of Sir Walter Running. Sandy was a phenom in his youth, and he's the fastest person I've ever known personally. He once ran a mile in a heartbreaking 4:01. When I talk about us fake *r-ugh-ners* versus those real *runners*, I am us and Sandy is them. However, I owe Sandy a huge debt. Back in 2019 when I was first building mileage for the Chicago Marathon, KT and I went to a wedding where we were seated next to Sandy and his wife. I talked to him about the marathon, and because I felt like a fraud talking about my slogging efforts to a guy who ran a sub-fourteen-minute 5K, I made a joke about the whole thing. I don't remember my joke because it was dumb and insecure and not really how I felt. What I remember is that Sandy didn't let the joke slide. He didn't even laugh to make me comfortable. He looked at me seriously and said, "Anyone who has gone out and experienced the pain of the road is a runner."

Yes.

That's how I felt. I was trying to do something hard. The running wasn't about what I could achieve. It was more entrenched. The running was about what I could overcome. There's a saying from Alcoholics Anonymous: "The only requirement for A.A. membership is the desire to stop drinking." All you need is want. I had that. I wanted to know what I was made of. I wanted to know if I could keep on going. Sandy understood, and he gave me an incredible gift that I hope you'll accept as well. It doesn't matter how far down the road you are. The victory is being out on the road. You could've stayed in, stayed online, stayed comfortable. You're experiencing the pain. That makes you a fellow traveler. And if you're doing your best on that road, you're not just traveling. You're running. That's me. Hi. I'm Dustin, and I'm a runner.

Sandy gave me that idea three years ago, and I've mostly shed my insecurities about pace and performance. Mostly. The part of me that wants to be better will always be a bit embarrassed about being slow, especially when contrasted with a running group like this one at the Raleigh Half preview. We take off at "easy" pace, and I run beside Sandy, chit-chatting about Bible study groups, mutual acquaintances, and I don't really know. Sandy is warming up, but we're running at an 8:30-minute-per-mile pace, so while Sandy's conversing, I'm doing math. This would be a 1:51:00 half marathon which would be my new PR. No chance. I tell Sandy I need to drop back. He already knew.

The course is an out-and-back. Two miles in, the main pack separates. A few miles later, when they pass me on the return, their running looks more like gliding, as if each step carries them twice as far as it's supposed to. Sandy dips down to set up a shin-level five, and he looks cool and at-ease. I do my best to mimic the vibe. We slap hands, and they're gone. My fellow travelers have left me behind. It feels both like freedom and a letdown. Mostly, it feels familiar. I realize this is the first time my mind has drifted since I began the run. I'm on my own. My pace is a steady 8:50 per mile. I'm tempted to turn on a podcast, or maybe Whitesnake's "Here I Go Again" to match the mood. But it's a beautiful day, and I'm extremely comfortable with my own mind. I am not bored.

If you find yourself bored when you run—if your mind is clamoring for distraction—you should find some people to run with. Anxiety thrives in solitude. Spend enough time with people who do what you're doing, and you'll stop registering the silliness of it all. Sharing the experience with others diminishes outside concerns and plunges your attention into the nuance of what's actually occurring in that window of time. Nothing changes about what you're doing except that someone else is doing it too, and for amateurs, that companionship is hugely therapeutic.

I'm on pace for a PR until about mile ten. Then cramps hit. My longest run since the knee injury was eight miles, and I did that at a ten-minute pace. The downside of running with others is sometimes you're so not-bored that you skip over the tedium of your own rules. I run faster and longer, and the consequences catch me before the finish line. This one time, it's really okay. I slow way down, walk-jog a couple more miles, and shuffle back to my car. Even though I'm dehydrated and achy, I also know for the first time in nearly three weeks that I'm normal. I have regular running problems. I get home, drop all my clothes on the floor, and make an Instagram post out of the heap. "Most importantly, my knee felt great. Time to build some volume."

I'm back! And by back, I mean in that struggling-to-run-a-solid-long-run kind of way! I'll see that course again in six weeks. The second half of this training is going to be tough and exhilarating. The long runs will creep up into the twenty-mile range, but also, I have two half-marathon races scheduled. The first one is in two weeks. The City of Oaks Half Marathon will be my first race in more than two years. I'm nervous, which is the same as excited. One surefire way to erase all boredom is to stop running and start racing.

Weeks 11 & 12
The City of Oaks Half Marathon

In week 11 of training for the Disney Marathon, I run thirty-eight miles with a long run of fifteen miles. I mix speed work into my five miles on Monday, including fast-slow intervals every 200m for twelve rounds. Then I cross-train with squats, core, pull-ups, and shoulder press. Tuesday is seven easy miles. Wednesday is six easy miles and core work. Thursday I do deadlifts, push-ups, and yoga, but I give running a rest. Friday we drive to Bluffton, SC to visit family. I run three easy upon arrival. Then I wake up the next morning and run fifteen miles. Sunday is two easy miles to recover. The long run isn't bad. My average pace for the run is just below ten minutes, and my heart rate never spikes. Still, I may have run the front end too fast. Ten miles seems to be a sticky point for me. That's when I feel signs of cramps. I slow down, eat a GU energy gel, and wonder if running with crossed fingers is a cute affectation. My body mostly holds, and I stiff leg the last couple of miles to finish. I should read the science about preventing cramps, but I used to cramp up at shorter distances. I tell myself that they'll go away as the body adapts to the training.

I don't think about those cramps really. Thirty-eight miles is my highest week of mileage in years. I'm happy. It's progress. Besides, week 12 is in my Monday morning coffee cup, and it fills my stomach with butterflies. There's a race on Saturday, the City of Oaks Half Marathon. KT is running too, and she's miserable about it.

While my knee, Row24, and the specter of cramping ruled my anxiety in the past few weeks, KT had her own training woes. She went out for a long run a few weeks back. Six miles in, she felt great, and in a thoughtless decision she will regret out loud a dozen times, she stopped to stretch her calves on a curb. It just happened. Maybe she anticipated a moment of relief that would mentally aid her through the back half of the run, but what she got was an immediate sense of discomfort. She tried to get back to stepping, but that discomfort turned to sharp pain, bad enough that she called me to bundle the kids into the car and pick her up. I housed my encouragement in practicality—time will tell, rest and revisit, blah blah blah—but KT had been running in some fashion for as long as I've known her, and this was the first call for a pickup I'd ever received. She tried running several times in the last few weeks. No dice. The calf issue was real, and ninety percent of her training transitioned to the Peloton Bike. Now, she has a half marathon on Saturday. She hasn't had a single good run in weeks. Her big hope is to finish.

For context, before pregnancy, KT routinely used half marathons as a fitness audit. If her mood waxed lazy or waned flabby, she'd put one on the schedule. Casual. A couple months of running, and she'd routinely run under 1:50 without any real nerves or trouble. To be worried about her body being able to simply finish a half was not only foreboding to the prospects of her first full marathon, but it was the exact opposite of the post-pregnancy strength reclamation she never really talks about. Under the skin, my wife is a harsh self-critic and fiery competitor. She commands these traits to her life's profit, but they don't always help her if forced to the surface. She hates being bad at things, and she hates people seeing her get pissy about being bad at those things. This is hilariously obvious when family members want to play board games she hasn't played before. She'd rather just not play. As if two pregnancies weren't enough, the calf injury is making her bad at running, and now the reckoning of a race is making that emotional burden heavier. She used to be able to do this. Is she still her or not? This running, this battle to repair and renew, it's not going well for either of us, and my methods of field dressing are not the same as hers. No matter the outcome, I'm confident in her ability to triage and keep her identity intact, but it would be so much easier if it just went well.

Then again, the reason we run is precisely because it is not easy. The effort is the reward.

Unlike KT, I enjoy putting my flaws on display. Sure, it's a controlled display. I don't have the strength of character to expose all my shittiness to the entire world. It took me a while to accept my limits, and it took me even longer to realize that discretionary sharing wasn't hypocrisy. The cliche is true: Discretion really is the better part of valor. It's courageous to share, but only share the thing you're actively working on. Have you ever scrubbed blood stains out of a shirt? It's cold water and soap before the stain sets. You pick a spot, scrub it like hell, and when you're satisfied, you go on to the next spot. Prioritize and execute. Trying to fix it all at once may be well intentioned, but it's foolish. This flaw I've put on display looks like it's about running, but it's really about discipline and consistency. It's about truly being who I say I am, and being able to do what I said I will do. On Monday, I post to Instagram the full week of what I'm going to do. Then I do it. At least, that's what I imply. But the runs are really secrets, aren't they? They happen (or not) when no one is looking. I'm self-reporting metrics. That's most weeks. Not this week. This week is a race, and a race is public. A race is a reckoning. I've claimed running as a priority. Can I execute? Or have I been a fool? Am I the master of my life, or am I a fraud?

I set my goals. They're humble, which is commentary on my low confidence. The A-goal is beating my only other half marathon time of 1:59:57. The B-goal is to finish. The C-goal is don't get injured.

My only other half was in San Diego in 2018. I was twenty-five pounds heavier, and it was the days of running hard and drinking harder. I was running with my older brother and his wife, Ava. KT was going to run, but she miscarried the day before we got on the plane to San Diego, and she just couldn't. The run started, and I sprinted out, leaving my brother and sister-in-law in the dust. My first mile was under eight minutes, then it continuously declined for the rest of the race, even as the last five miles were entirely downhill. Somewhere around mile eleven, my phone rang. I looked and saw "Joe Riedesel." If something had happened to my brother, it would have to wait. I was dying on the road, limping to a miserable finish, but I had to finish before I could think about anything else. I hit ignore, and as I did, I looked up to see my brother jogging beside me with his cell phone to his ear.

"Ignore!?" He smiled through a face of mock hurt.

My older brother. He looked fresh. He also looked like a jolly ghost haunting my teenage insecurities. Still, I was glad to see him. Ava was with him, and she was basically dance-running my pace with wired headphones jacked into a handheld phone. I felt ridiculous. I felt pain. I felt regret for setting this goal of a sub-two-hour half and ignoring all the things I needed to do to achieve it. But Joe and Ava didn't care about all that. They didn't even care about their own pace. The end of the half curved around corners of downtown San Diego. Joe would run ahead to the corner and linger, looking back and waving me in, making sure I didn't walk. He knew it was close, and he did this at four or five corners until we saw the finish line at mile 13.1. Technically, that race was a success, and I'll always be grateful to my family for carrying me through it. Inside though, I felt silly. I'd been a hypocrite for a while, and I felt exposed by the race. My body was broken for the week following. There were four full days of limping everywhere I went as my feet and ankles slowly mended themselves back together. It's the worst I've ever felt after a run.

So that's what KT and I have in our heads as we wake up on race-day Saturday morning. We're nervous, but that's a good thing. Ken Rideout won the Myrtle Beach Marathon at age fifty-one. He spoke about pre-race jitters on the Bare Performance Podcast saying, "Yeah, of course you're nervous. Cause it matters. And you care. And it's time." We start the coffee, make our oatmeal with honey, almond butter, and bananas, and try to hydrate early enough to pee our bladders back to peaceful before go-time. Her parents are there to watch the kids as we shuffle out the front door.

The City of Oaks is a nice size race, hosting a couple thousand runners. KT and I are dragging a cauldron of anxiety into this race, but we also carry two clean aces. The first ace is a starting line that sits less than a half-mile from our front door. It is a blessing to avoid the hassles of transportation, parking, gear check, and everything else involved in proper race-day planning. We just walk out our front door and join the parade of people migrating to the corrals. For this reason alone, I will run something between the 5K and full marathon with City of Oaks for as long as I live in my current home. The second ace is the course itself. It is comprised entirely of roads we cover every week in our daily training. It's not an easy course, but we know it cold. Speaking of cold, it's forty-three degrees to start the race, and will be mid-fifties by the time we finish. That's perfect since we can just walk out, warm-up, and run.

KT and I take a pre-race picture and wish each other luck. I'm trying to PR. She's just hoping for a pain-free run. I'll meet her at the finish line.

I feel incredible in the first two miles. I remember a quote I saw on the @RunningExplained Instagram. A 2:20 marathoner named Sarah Hall said, "It's amazing how the same pace in practice can seem so much harder than on race day. Stay confident. Trust the process." I feel like I'm barely trying in these first two miles. In fact, I am consciously telling myself to stay slow. Slow down. I don't want to repeat my hot start mistake from San Diego. "Nice and easy, Dust." I'm borderline fanatical about staying chill. All this effort to be slow; I look at my pace for mile one. 8:33. Stay chill. I look at mile two. 8:38.

The course breaks from downtown and enters into some rolling hills through neighborhoods, but I know these hills. "Chill up the hill," I repeat in mind. I know I'll make it up on the descents. Mile three is 8:36. Mile four is 8:38.

The next two miles are key, a massive descent followed by a massive climb on Ashe Avenue. I've been using a smallish, fit-looking fellow as a makeshift pacer, staying a couple yards off him. We hit the descent and he begins to fly forward. I'm tempted to kick in with him, but I know that Ashe is the toughest hill of the entire course, and it is coming up in mile six. Ashe is the quarter-mile hill I run for repeats on a weekly basis. I know how it will deplete my gas tank. I let the pacer gap me. I'll find someone else. I grab a gel and use the descent to hold pace in active recovery. Mile five is 8:30.

There's a mostly flat stretch on Western Blvd before the Ashe hill where I fall into pace beside a couple that seem very intense on holding their current effort. I feel my first real battle with my ego, and it surfaces some ugly mental chatter. *I'm fitter than these schmucks. He's doughy, and look at her legs flail outward with each stride. They're not athletes. They're not runners.* I feel bad even as I think it, but it's no time to judge my brain. The chatter is a sign that my mind has been tagged into the fight, and it's explaining to me—albeit vindictively—why I can do this. I'm in the middle third of the race, and I'm experiencing the race's effect on human experience in real time. The first third of a race is physical. The second third is physical and mental. The last third will be physical, mental, and emotional.

We hit Ashe. With no curves or trees to obstruct full view of its climb, the hill is basically talking trash. Some runners lean in, some start to walk. My pace couple of the last mile continues to hold pace, gritting their teeth and gapping me. My ego recoils at the separation, but I say it again, "Chill up the hill." I focus on attaching my effort to my heart rate and keeping it as even as the Western Boulevard flat. The climb feels longer than usual. My legs are burning by the time I reach the top, but my lungs are okay. I feel the lactic acid dissipate from my quads as the road flattens out. Mile six is 9:22.

Mile seven and eight run down Hillsborough Street through the campus of North Carolina State University. I'd been laser focused on not crushing myself during the big Ashe climb, and my plan was to make up pace now. Maybe it's because I run Hillsborough multiple times a week, but I'd blocked out how hilly it actually is. For the first time ever, I find myself considering the etymology of the word. Hills. Borough. A town set in the hills. Maybe this isn't the best road to make up pace. I'm getting tired. Mile seven is 8:57. Mile eight is 9:04.

The song "Revelry" by Kings of Leon thrums in my ears. My heart is in my throat, and grenades of passionate regrets feel as destructive as they did ten years ago. *What the hell is going on*, I think, and I realize it's the last third of the race. Emotion has joined my brain and body to finish the fight. I force an audible laugh to embrace the chaos. Mile nine is 8:39.

My inner thigh twitches, and my whole body shocks cold with fear. A cramp? *No, no, no. Not now. It's too soon.* I shorten my stride, I walk through the next aid station as I double fist Powerade. I take a deep breath to clear the emotion and find my mind. It doesn't work. I keep moving. I'm deep inside, almost angry at my own body. *Who do you* think *is in charge here?* More encouraging as the steps normalize; *we got this.* I'm nearly oblivious to the outside world until I notice the chorus to "I Hold On" by Dierks Bentley is in my headphones. It feels like providence. This song and thoughts of Walter carried me during the final mile of the Chicago marathon. I think of my son now, which is the most gracious way I can think of myself. How will he respond in those difficult moments when he's afraid he might not ever be the man he hopes to become? I think about how I hope he sees me, and I think about how I hope, impossibly, that he thinks I'm the best man he's ever known even as I know that he's a much better man than I ever was. The dad-insanity is raging, and I might even be crying while I'm running, but I'm also not cramping. I'm not cramping at all. I feel strong. I'm preparing myself for a push with meaningless phrases like, "Only you, Riedesel. Only you, Dust." I'm not sure what it means, but I heard David Goggins say it to himself in an audiobook once and it makes me feel like a damn grizzly bear. Why that feeling helps me run, who knows. But I'm fading, so I'll use anything that keeps me moving. Near the end of mile ten, I'm turning back onto Hillsborough Street for the return trip to the finish line. My head is looking through my feet into a well of self-motivation when a voice through my headphones snaps me upright.

"Dust! Dustin!"

KT is waving, running the opposite direction, turning off Hillsborough as I turn onto it. I clumsily pump a fist above my head or something, trying to come back to reality, but I don't have anything to say, really. She does, and it's exactly what I need to here.

"Walter is at David's Dumplings!"

Okay, David's Dumplings is about a mile and a half down Hillsborough. My body is either going to hold on or it won't, but when Walter looks at me, there won't be any question. I'm going to be *running*. Mile ten was 9:12. Mile eleven is 8:11.

My Half Marathon Playlist on Spotify ends. All good. Ain't nothin' gonna break my stride. I tap twice on my headphones to restart it, but that's not how all my stuff is wired apparently. My Apple Music app starts and plays the first file it has, a song called "Bluegrass" by a Christian rapper named Trav. I played basketball with Trav in college, and I buy all his albums because being creative is a hard effort that deserves support. It's not my first choice of running music, but the song builds to a crescendo with a driving beat, and Trav pours his heart into bars of a little boy growing up to discard personal demons and find purpose in his Heavenly Father. The vibes are close enough. I let it repeat as I run hard to finish. On the way, I pass the intense pace couple who separated from me on the hill. My competitiveness and arrogance are gone. I only feel a sense of connection to their effort, and I'm proud of us both.

Walter is with KT's dad outside David's Dumplings. Walter is pumped to see me, and KT's dad has a big smile. I slow down to give out fist bumps. The delay is worth it. Mile twelve is 7:54.

And that's it. I've already won. Midway through the mile, Trav starts singing "Bluegrass" for the third time, and I can't believe I have so much energy in a thirteenth mile. As I get into the downtown finish line, I run around four or five corners, and no one's waving me in, but something's pulling me in. Mile thirteen is 7:12.

Mile 0.1 is 6:32.

That's a new half PR of 1:52:39.

A few minutes later, the pace couple runs across the line in a sub-two-hour effort. The girl is crying, but they're both happy.

"Dusty!"

I look up and see my friend Mike Mabunga. He ran the race too, finishing with a PR of his own at 1:37. I'm on too much of a high to feel even an ounce of jealousy; I'm simply impressed.

"I just hung on to the 1:40 pacer and then went for it at the end," he says.

Running with a real pacer? I make a mental note.

Mike hangs out and we wait for KT. She crosses around the 2:20 mark. It's the slowest half marathon of her life, but I can tell she's feeling what I felt during the Half Preview a couple weeks prior. Her calf didn't hurt her at all. She can run again!

The three of us eat our bananas and collect the post-race swag as we excitedly share stories from inside the race. Apparently Walter ran out into the middle of the race to hug KT as she ran by. KT's dad captured a video of it that I watch later, and as I write this, it's still a top-five video clip in my memories. Mike agrees to come on the *Looks Like We're Lost* podcast the following week and really nerd out about the whole race. We have a happy farewell and KT and I walk back home.

And that's the race. It's a microcosm of the whole running experience. Fear, hope, struggle, companionship, isolation, perseverance, and ultimately the sense of peace that comes when you realize the effort is the reward. When you run a race well, the excitement you feel is multi-faceted, but it is more anticipatory than conclusive. The accomplishment is self-discovery. It's a factual experience about who you are now and who you are becoming. The reward is not simply that you finished. It's that you are certain you can do it all again. You ran.

Congratulations.

You get to run some more.

Week 13
The Photo Package

Analyzing the training efforts is a continuous process. However, the majority of reflection happens after a race. You have your time, your medal, a head full of glorious memories, and an overpriced packet of digital photographs to consider buying. How do those pictures make you feel?

One of the oddities about running is that most of us have no idea how we look when we run. I cannot see myself running, and no matter how awkward my running motion may appear, it is the most natural movement in the world. Most of us amateurs haven't refined our form; we just run however we run, and this makes us especially vulnerable to photography. After a race, the event organizers send out thousands of photos sorted by bib number or facial recognition. It's a cash grab, but it's also a chance to relive the thrills! Who amongst the running community has not clicked on the race-day photo links with naive eagerness, aching to see a picture that captures our peak strength and athleticism as we triumph over the road? We click through picture after picture. There's too much lens flare. The camera angle is obstructed by other runners. We're not in the picture at all. Finally, a clear shot catches us in a short stride, or our eyes are closed, or we're hunched over, trudging up a hill. We click some more, but there are no more pictures with us in them.

There are three good running pictures of me ever. Maybe. More like one good picture and two that don't need to be flagged for sensitive content. They're fine. They're notable for what they're not.

No grimacing, no walking, no beet-red face. They're pictures of a guy not suffering while also not moving at his slowest speed. I should frame them in platinum with a black opal plate that reads, "Picture rarer than the frame."

Related: I saw a video on Instagram that I love. In it, a mom runs with a stroller. She's moving fast, and the music is something like "Can't Hold Us" by Macklemore & Ryan Lewis. The camera moves smooth and fluid like her stride, staying right beside her while holding her footsteps and the stroller's spinning tires in perfect balance on the lower third of the frame. Then there's a jump cut. We're watching from the outside perspective of someone on a porch. The picture immediately looks amateurish, which is to say it looks authentic, and there's no music bed. The only effect is some lens flare from a pleasant sunrise in a standard American suburb. The woman and the stroller are rolling down the street, but the pace seems very average from this viewpoint. Beside the woman is a man on a bicycle, barely pedaling, holding a digital camera on a gimbal. I gave the image a heart and considered a comment. Maybe quote Aristotle: "The aim of art is not to represent the outward appearance of things, but their inward significance." Maybe quote Picasso: "Art is a lie that makes us realize the truth." Maybe quote a t-shirt I saw once: "The Earth without Art is just Eh." In the end, no comment. I just share the post with KT because art is meant to be shared, then I leave it alone until this paragraph.

What's the point of all this? Am I driving at something specific with all this photo package talk? Is this book called *Looks Like We're Photographed*? Is that Nickelback's music stuck in my head now? Let's keep going.

In week 13 of training for the Disney Marathon, I do not run forty-one miles with a long run of seventeen miles. That was the plan, but I fail miserably. I run six miles on Tuesday, then fly to Kentucky to visit friends. Upon landing, I run eight miles. I am supposed to run ten miles the next morning, but I stay up until almost four in the morning drinking beer and talking about God and family and the metaphorical essence undergirding every form of human communication. *Dude, I'm telling you, the only way to know something without metaphor is to be present in the experience, man, before it's been tainted by memory and explanation.* That is not wrong, so I won't try to explain how much ass I feel like when I wake up five hours later. I put on my shoes. Ten miles is on the calendar. I run two, then sit on a curb in downtown Lexington and stare into the cement for five minutes.

What am I doing here?

I go back to the hotel. My friends are still sleeping. I take a shower, get dressed, push all thoughts of guilt and self-deception out of my mind, and I don't run for the rest of the week. I fly home on Saturday morning.

KT and I don't have a lot of rules. We understand each other, I think, and we're extremely communicative about what we're feeling and planning. She might actually like it if I shared a little less. But one rule I have for myself is to not intentionally lie to KT about anything. If I can't tell her the truth, then I don't have good reasons for doing what I'm doing, and if I don't have good reasons, then I shouldn't be doing them. Creating a good life is about wisdom, strength and kindness. Choose to want the right things (wisdom), pursue them doggedly (strength), and treat yourself and others with empathy along the way (kindness). My strength and kindness have always been decent. I'm not lazy or cruel. But I need KT for wisdom. She provides me an honesty and accountability that guides my wanting. In that way, she completes me. Hence the rule to not lie. Well, I realized I've done a pretty good job of following that rule because when I get home, I am rusty. KT just looks at me, and she knows.

"Did you drink?" KT asks. I say no. I just stayed up late. I'm tired, but I'm fine. I'm going to go do my long run now so I can hit my mileage and relax. She says ok because that's all she needs to say. There's no jury to win over. I was supposed to run seventeen miles. I run eleven, stop, put my hands on my hips and just stare at the sky.

What am I doing here?

I jog home and apologize. I ask for forgiveness. We talk through it. She forgives me. I guess it's fine. My drinking issues have always been about losing self-control. I drank, and I didn't embarrass myself. I didn't paint the town. I had drinks while catching up with some of my closest friends, and I laughed more in three days than I usually do in a month. By almost anyone's standards, there is nothing to be ashamed of. Even me with all my drinking-related issues, I don't believe drinking is wrong. I only believe alcohol is unhealthy and potentially dangerous, and I need more control than most. The whole week was a loss of self-control. I said I'd do something, and I didn't. Then I lied. If I was telling myself to not feel guilty, the lie confirmed that I *was* guilty. Maybe I shouldn't feel ashamed, but I definitely feel guilty. The guilt is a silver lining, actually. Choosing to want the right things is also a continuous process.

Something I've learned running: All the runs are connected. You're welding links on a chain, and if every run is an A-plus link, the chain will be strong enough to pull you through race day. Equally important, the chain will be strong enough to make you proud of your handiwork. You will look at what you have made, and it will be very good. The longer the race, the longer chain you need, and it is more difficult to make enough quality links. Running twenty-seven miles instead of forty-one isn't enough links. Running thirteen of those twenty-seven miles hungover, dehydrated, and travel-worn isn't enough quality. I didn't make many quality links when my knee was hurt, but it's easy to forgive that. This week 13, though? It's shit handiwork. Even if this training chain is strong enough to pull me through the Disney Marathon at my desired pace, I'm going to always be annoyed by this malformed link where I didn't do what I said I would. And me and KT? Well, I'm fortunate that there are two people crafting our relationship links. Forgiveness can turn some poor handiwork into something strong. KT is gracious, and I do believe she trusts me where it counts, trusts my intentions, my net positive. I've heard some people talk about their spouses forging a whole string of unwanted links. "The old ball and chain." That's not been my experience. KT and I are not responsible for each other's feelings, and I don't drag around some heavy, twisted idea of marriage. But I am responsible for my actions, and in a marriage, I'm responsible for matching my words to those actions. The consistency with which I actually do what I said I would do—that predictability—is real trust. That's how one becomes trustworthy.

So, about that photo package. Those photos aren't lies. If I look slow in twenty-nine of thirty photos, I doubt it's some conspiracy from the billionaires behind Big Race Photo. The reason I look slow is because I'm comparing those twenty-nine photos to every running photo I've ever seen, and everyone else on the planet who has ever posted a photo of their running has posted photo thirty, not the slow twenty-nine. Photo thirty sells shoes. Photo thirty goes up on social media. Photo thirty is the shiniest link in the chain, and it's the only part of the chain we see when we look at others.

What does any of this have to do with running? I was going to write this later, but I'll write it now. No one will ever care about you as much as you care about yourself. Maybe you have some guilt about something and you just carry it around. Well, guilt is just the beginning of self-care. If you can realize that care is actually love, that even the things you feel the worst about are shadows cast by love, then you can understand what all this has to do with running. Can I turn my weak and tired body into something strong and resilient? Can I endure? Running is about figuring out how to do something difficult. It's about peace of mind. It's about how consistency equates to success. Solve the addiction or don't. Run the miles or don't. Break four hours or don't. Grand scheme of things, no one will care. No one but you. "Only you, Riedesel." I used to think the argument of right versus wrong was about consequences, but outcome alone isn't enough to understand right and wrong. The argument of right versus wrong is a question of identity. There will always be a photo thirty, a moment that stands out from the rest. What makes photo thirty hypocritical—or not—is something only you will know in your heart of hearts. One link in your life will always be the strongest, sure, but if you've poured care and attention into every link, then you'll have no shame in pointing to any length of the chain. You'll be proud to display any photo in the packet. Heck, you'll be proud with nothing to display at all. You will love yourself. You will love even the parts that you feel the worst about. You will have peace of mind.

It's going to be hard for me to not regret this twenty-seven-mile week that should've been forty-one, but I've been kind to myself. I've done all I can to turn my poor handiwork into something strong. The next step is simple. Keep going.

Weeks 14 & 15
The Holiday Runs

Oh, the holidays. A wonderful and trying time for any family, but for parents who run, there are extra considerations. KT and I will be traveling two weekends in a row, a cross-state drive to visit her family *before* Thanksgiving, and a flight to Austin, Texas to visit my family *on* Thanksgiving. Two weeks on the road makes it tougher to get out on the road.

We'll manage, but first, a tip to all the new parents out there. Buy direct flights. It's what, an extra six hundred doll hairs? That doesn't even mean anything. What's meaningful is eliminating stress, decreasing the potential for chaos, and minimizing the exhaustion of entertaining a toddler in a terminal without melting their retinas—and their curiosity—with an endless amount of brighter-than-the-real-world, let-me-think-for-you, screen-time babysitting. When we visit my parents in Kansas City, there are no direct flights, and I always consider driving two hours from Raleigh to Charlotte to fly direct. I never do it and spend every moment languishing in the overstuffed seating bay of a Hartsfield-Jackson, a Dulles International, or occasionally, inexplicably, a Philadelphia International, wondering if I'd be happier driving to my more expensive direct flight in Charlotte.

Whatever. *C'est la vie.* Holidays are tricky. Even if you do everything in your power to simplify, the holidays add some stressors.

In week 14 of training for the Disney Marathon, I run forty-two

miles with a long run of seventeen miles. This severely violates my
rule of no more than a ten percent increase week over week, but
given my failure to log miles last week, I have to increase my risk
profile. There isn't a ton of time between now and Disney. So I run
seven miles on Monday, doing three sets of 1.5-mile tempo runs in
the middle; then I cross-train squats, push-ups, and pull-ups. I run
ten easy miles on Tuesday, cross-training shoulders and arms. I run
six miles with hill intervals on Wednesday, cross-training deadlifts
and core. I don't run Thursday, but I ride the Peloton, do push-ups,
pull-ups, and more core.

I am sufficiently crushed in the first half of the week, and not just
physically. Tuesday, I leave the house in standard running attire. I
like to run shirtless, but Tuesday is chilly enough to merit a t-shirt
and gloves. I'm running a familiar route when I feel some churning
in my gut. It isn't long before this churning graduates into a full-
blown, intestinal Chernobyl. Put five minutes on the Doomsday
Clock. Am I mixing metaphors? My history on nuclear disaster is
itself a disaster. Here's some history I do know. The last time I shit
my pants while running was a coach-pitch baseball game when I
six. It inspired a friend to sing a charming ditty about pooping
myself as I rounded the bases:

When you're running down to first,
And your pants are gonna burst, diarrhea
When you're sliding into second,
And you feel something peckin', diarrhea

Third-turd. Home-foam. You get it. Kids are diabolical. It was a
devastating limerick, not just because I was the victim, the one
literally and figuratively shat on, but because it was hilarious. It
rhymed. It was catchy. In more ways than one, the burn was acidic.

I'd rather not poop my pants again. Maybe I hadn't given it a lot
of thought, but up until this very moment, I was optimistic about
hitting the thirtieth year of my non-shitting-myself-while-running
streak. Now it's all in jeopardy. I'm three miles from home. No

chance. I'm in a midtown neighborhood at 10:00 a.m. on a weekday. Do I knock on doors and beg for toilet access? Do I duck into a backyard? There has to be better way. I'm looking desperately for some of those randomly stationed "they poop, you scoop" doggy bags. If I do have to drop my pants and a load in the public view, maybe I'll be forgiven because I did the civil thing and picked up my mess. Good Lord in heaven, the veil of civility is so thin, isn't it? When facing self-defecation, your brain scrambles like a caged animal. I take a deep breath. I know there's a construction zone in three-quarters of a mile. Gut-check time, Riedesel. I squeeze the cheeks and try some controlled breathing. Pace is *ppphhhtt*, occurring, I guess. Focus on the porta-potty. Nothing exists but the porta-potty. It's a good plan until it's not. The downside of becoming singularly minded is that when the Doomsday Clock hits zero, I don't have contingencies. I'm coming up on a church. Kids are playing outside. Exposure is nigh at this house of the Lord, but illegal indecency is not my main concern. The kids are about six years old—prime limerick age—and I can already hear a chorused remix of the diarrhea song, gospel edition. Just as I'm thinking my Lord has abandoned me and closed every door, he opens a window. I speed-waddle over a three way stop, press my hands into a prayer emoji and wedge-dive into a tall and *probably* opaque set of hedges. I get deep. Completely hidden. I'm in a cold sweat of panic and desperation as the feces surges towards my butt cheeks. My hands are shaking so badly and moving so quickly that I'm not sure my shorts have cleared the drop zone. It doesn't matter. Relief washes away the fear. I'm baptized in acceptance. This will just be what it is.

And it is natural. I clear my chamber. I clear my shorts. It is finished. All that's left is a choice. Do I sacrifice the gloves or the shirt? I choose shirt, hoping the resourceful Mother Nature can make use of my donation. Emerging from the hedge, I lock eyes with a dump truck sitting at the stop. The driver stares at me with no expression whatsoever, and I run away. I run past the kids without giving them a glance. I just run home. When I get there, KT asks, "How'd your run go?" I say it went well. She wrinkles her forehead. "Weren't you wearing a shirt?"

When hiding in church shrubbery at mid-morning to empty your bowels isn't the low point of your last seven days, you need to talk to someone. We're in Hickory, NC for my Friday easy run, and there's an Alcoholics Anonymous meeting three miles from KT's parents' house. I have KT drop me there so I can run back after. It's hard to imagine a better way to care for myself in only ninety minutes.

Looks Like We're Running is not about addiction recovery, except that it is. Something a twelve-step program teaches you is that the only way to overcome a desire is with a greater desire. Denial is not effective. Your appetite abhors a vacuum. If you are trying to convince yourself that running is something you could get into, there's a reason. Maybe you are overweight. Maybe you are trying to recover health after an injury or a sickness or a pregnancy. Maybe you are afflicted by regretful personal decisions and just running to feel some control. Maybe you are running away from something, but also, you are running towards something. You are running towards health. You are running towards a clear mind and an energized body. You are running towards yourself, and this version of you is present. You are a thoughtful person, a patient person, and a person who can say the words "yes" and "no" without guilt. The most important word in any of these scenarios is "you." Only you really know why you are running and who you are running towards. Like anyone, your reasons are unique, but that doesn't mean they should be secrets. The thing I learned simultaneously about runners and addicts is that they're all people. No matter how tempting it is to put people into stereotypical boxes, they don't *actually* fit. People are not ideas. If we occasionally share a room, a coffee, a stretch of road, then that camaraderie is a gift, but it isn't our identity. All people are different people. Your reasons for showing up on the road or in a meeting are exactly what they need to be. And if I ever see you there, I promise no judgment, only grace and gratitude.

I look like a tourist in this particular AA meeting. I'm wearing bright orange running shoes. I have a short-brimmed Rogue running cap. It's also Friday at noon, and the average age of the meeting is roughly twenty-five years my senior. Most are regulars. They obviously know each other, even if it's *only* on a first-name basis. The hour is endearing and heartbreaking. Thanksgiving is next week, and many share stories of estranged children they still aren't allowed to see, grandkids they've never met, and how they'll be celebrating a meager, solitary thanksgiving in which their biggest chunk of gratitude comes from still being alive and being sober. Some stories are told with humor, some with remorse, but none are a surprise. Anyone who has gone out and experienced the pain of self-destruction knows these stories. It's nice we have each other. When it comes to me, I share my gratitude for the group, that there are places for crash-landings, and for the stupid luck that I crashed before my kids were born. To myself, I promise to not take Thanksgiving with my family for granted. A few shares later, a woman breaks down in tears. Her brother died of an overdose only three weeks ago. She's wretched from guilt. Should she have been there with him? At the end of the meeting she picks up her chip for being one-year sober. I don't pick up a chip. That's not my way. But I feel stronger, more myself. We're all running our own race, and though my progress is slow, my pace is steady. For no reason in particular, I listen to "Nightswimming" by REM as the first song on my jog back to KT's parents' house. The song isn't really about anything, except maybe a personal experience, and maybe the appreciation of that experience.

You, I thought I knew you
You I cannot judge

You, I thought you knew me

With grandparents watching the kids, KT and I run seventeen miles together the next day. It takes three hours. Hickory is nestled in the foothills of the Appalachian Mountains, so this is a tough seventeen, but also, it's not. We take it slow. We hang in there. The time is the effort. KT and I never get to run together, and having someone to talk to makes the run way better. We talk about the kids, the future, our own issues, and by time this rare, three hours of unbroken conversation is finished, the tension from the prior week feels far away. There is something experiential to share in seventeen miles. Resolve, endurance, commitment, and sacrifice turn an arbitrary distance into a meaningful time. It's not romance exactly, but it is love, and I'm glad we're doing it together.

In week 15 of training for the Disney Marathon, I run forty-three miles with a long run of nineteen miles. I run seven Fartlek miles on Monday, followed by easy miles of six and eight on Tuesday and Wednesday. My cross training is brief, only doing compound lifts for a few sets after the runs. Squats on Monday. Deadlifts on Tuesday. They're light. I'm just trying to keep the joints loose. We fly to Austin and have a great Thanksgiving. The smoked turkey is so superior to the baked turkey that I decide then and there my next book will be unfortunately titled *Looks Like We're Smoking* to chronicle the amateur pursuit of eating delicious meats. I run three miles on Friday, and if I thought Texas was going to be flat, then I thought wrong. The neighborhood is one of the hilliest I've seen not nestled in the mountains. I'm extremely worried about Saturday's nineteen miles.

Fortunately, my older brother runs a decent amount. At six feet, 230 pounds, he's not primarily an endurance athlete, but he's not afraid of long distance. He's run a marathon. He also took second in the Clydesdale's division of a half Ironman. For those unfamiliar, that's 1.2 miles swimming, fifty-six miles biking, then a 13.1-mile run. I'm confident in my brother's recommendation. He places us on a fairly flat out-and-back. It's difficult, but we finish every last step of nineteen miles. I'm mostly just relieved that I have KT for these last two long runs. It's a good reminder at this time of year. The best thing about family holidays isn't the holiday.

Next week is a de-load week that ends with a half-marathon race, and I find myself feeling a new sensation. I'm actually relieved that a half-marathon is such a short distance.

Week 16
The Raleigh Half: "Go Get It"

Here's something I would like to change in my writing: I use the word "it" too frequently. "It" sounds splendid to the writer, because to the writer, it is splendid. It is a feeling, and the writer is so incredibly close to it. He knows what "it" refers to, and it refers to it perfectly and in totality. The writer can see how it details each photon of difference between lightning and the lightning bug. "It" is the perfect metaphor, relaying all the vibes the writer has vibed. "It" can say anything, which is why I've used it often. Such is my shame. Because "it" only occasionally says the precise thing. I would not be surprised if Stephen King's inspiration for the novel *It* came from editing out insecure pronouns in his own second drafts. The titular "It" is Pennywise, a demon clown described as an evil, shapeshifting entity that preys on the fear of its victims. That's what "it" feels like to me: insecurity made manifest. Abandon this pronoun, young writer. It will only cause chaos.

Then again, what if I want to embrace the chaos? What if I need to be open to anything in order to press forward? Well, I can think of a few perfectly meaningless phrases that get great results.

Bring it on.

Just do it.

Go get it.

You know those first two. They led to a great movie and a great marketing campaign. And that last one? Well, that's what this chapter is about.

When marathon training, is it good to build some shorter races like the half marathon into the training plan? Physically speaking, no one can say. The science is beyond us, and by "us," I'm talking about the population too lazy to Google the science. Forget the science. Let me tell you something that's beyond the science. Running half marathons during your marathon training is the ballz. With a "z." Prove me wrong, science! You can't. As with all plurals ending in z, the data is anecdotal.

In week 16 of training for the Disney Marathon, I run thirty-five miles, with a long run of 13.1 miles. I squat and ride Peloton on Monday. I run seven Fartlek miles (these are miles where you constantly vary your intensity by mixing up the pace or terrain) and deadlift on Tuesday. Ten easy miles on Wednesday. Three easy miles on Friday. Fifteen miles on Saturday with a warm-up and cool-down rounding out the half.

I'm wearing new shoes. The shoes feel huge. Not physically huge, but metaphorically. They are taking up a ton of my mental real estate. The shoes are the Nike ZoomX Vaporfly Next% 2 if we're being precise. They're white with neon trim in leukemia-awareness orange and secure-in-my-masculinity pink. They look hot. They look fast. They look like something a real runner would wear, and I feel simultaneously cool as hell and fraudulent as shit. I'm faking it, yes, but I'm also confident, because I might be on my way to making it. There's a bounce in my step, and it's mostly the shoes, but it's partially my belief in the shoes. Running gurus I've listened to say, "Nothing new on race day." And I'm abiding by that rule because I ran three easy miles in these shoes the day before, so the newness is not one hundred percent new. Totally acceptable. The rest of race-day's ensemble includes my participant, dri-fit t-shirt from the Chicago Marathon, five-inch Under Armor Speedpocket shorts, a Rogue running cap, Goodr sunglasses, Balega quarter socks, AirPods, and an Apple Watch with a freshly downloaded playlist. All of that attire was incorporated naturally. It feels right. But the shoes feel gaudy, ostentatious. Am I overcompensating?

Have I worn a tuxedo to the job interview?

I've found the 1:50 pace flag, and I'm going to hang with that group for a new PR. The Raleigh Half is hosted by Sir Walter Running on the Raleigh Greenway. The Greenway is an eight-foot-wide strip of pavement that snakes through the entire city. The pace group alleviates my nerves about navigating runners on such a narrow course. If I'm lucky, I'll have some gas in the tank at the end to get under the 1:50 time. When it comes to PR times, the further a number is to the left, the more pride there is in flipping it down another digit. This is why breaking the hour-length barriers are the most treasured. But right after the hours, every ten-minute barrier you can crush is like holy water from the fountain of youth being fresh-squeezed into your mouth. That imagery might not work for you. Fair enough, but trust me. Seeing a one-fifty-anything become a one-forty-anything is where the "z" in "ballz" comes from.

My breakfast, parking, warm-up, and pee break have all timed out perfectly. I'm at the starting line with zero concerns and only a couple GU Energy Gels in my pocket. The cramps from this course's preview run six weeks prior are on the edges of my mind, but even with that bad week in the middle, the past six weeks have made me better. I'm ready. Then I hear counting into a bullhorn as I naturally drift forward with the herd. I start my watch, and the race has begun.

The 1:50 pacer is a guy—let's call him Pacey—and he is wearing a short-sleeve, button-up shirt with floral print. His stride is as casual as his attire. This is my first pacer ever, and the vibes are easy. To Pacey, this race is a day at the beach, so that's how he dressed. After a half mile, I look at my watch and do math in my head, but it's purely a curiosity. My trust in Pacey is complete. Mile one is 8:05.

The preview run from six weeks prior pays dividends. As a big guy, hills take an extra toll on me. Pacey pulls our group up a steep hill faster than I like. I let them separate, knowing that I can catch up on the longer slope of the backside. Mile two is 8:11.

Similar to the City of Oaks, I feel the initial energy of the race dissipate in the third mile. Now I feel steady. The strength and confidence are there, and I feel connected to my body, not like I'm elevated by a high. Mile three is 8:03.

By my math, we're a little hot. Pacey must realize it too. He dials us back a smidge. Miles four through eight run 8:11, 8:15, 8:19, 8:18, and 8:18. During this middle section, our pace group dwindles from about twenty-five runners to five. For those not able to hang with Pacey's leisurely trot, the drop off is evenly dispersed. We seem to lose someone every five minutes. But the most concentrated loss for the group isn't folks falling off. We make the turn on this out-and-back at mile seven, and over the next mile, something like ten runners turn it up to leave Pacey and pals behind. I stay with the pals, and I wonder what made folks decide to break this early. Is upping pace at the halfway mark a good strategy? Did seeing the elite runners sprinting by after their turn fuel ambitions? Maybe some runners who were cautious on the out feel confident on the back now that they've covered the course? I don't know, but each departure has me feeling the itch to turn it up.

Finishing this race above a sustainable pace is tricky. I make a quick analysis of the possibilities. I have five miles left. My fastest recorded five miles were back in week 4. I ran it at a 7:35 pace. Could I hold that now? I was fresh when I ran that. Matching that PR with eight miles already on the treads would be a tall task. What would cover the fatigue gap of those eight miles? I have the shoes. I have race-day vibes. I have twelve weeks of training, eight-and-a-half of them quality. Is that enough? Maybe. Analyze the risk. What am I afraid of? I don't want to lose a PR. That's all. Anything else is outside of race scope. The only way I lose the PR is cramps, my old nemesis, and that fear informs my compromise. I have one more GU gel in my pocket, and I know we're passing an aid station near the end of the ninth mile. That's where I'll dig in. I'll take the GU in slowly, get some fluid at the station, then I'll run the last four miles hard. It's settled. Mile nine is 8:20.

After the aid station, I pat Pacey on the back. I've been behind him for the entirety of the last nine miles, and I think this is the first time he's seen me all day. It doesn't matter. I'm thanking him for *me*. Gratitude to others is a gift to yourself. And I'm so glad I gave myself that gift, because if I hadn't, then I would never had heard Pacey say what he says.

I say, "Hey man, thanks for getting me here."

Pacey says, "Go get it."

"It" is perfect. Mile ten is 7:21.

I pass a couple of the early breakers from Pacey's group, and I feel good about my choice to hold off. This next mile has the steepest ascent of my return, but it's not too long. I take it as fast as I can without tapping the tank. I pass two of the early breakers from Pacey's group who are walking to finish the rise. I hold the ascent pace for about ten seconds after reaching the top. *Enough rest, Dust. Go get it.* Mile eleven is 7:37.

The next mile is gentle, rolling hills. I find myself wondering if I could've run the whole race this way. The first eight miles felt like shuffling compared to my current stride. Like justice for training, I bend arcs around the strugglers of this stretch run, and a question pops into my head: Is this how *runners* get to feel? There's only one way to answer the question, and I'm getting it. I smile to myself and imagine waiting for Pacey at the finish line just to tell him that I got it. I almost laugh out loud because no, I won't do that. Would Pacey understand? Then I do laugh, like a crazy person. This is the real runner's high. It's all vibes. I decide to give up ten to fifteen seconds to stop at an aid station. It's probably a mistake, and even now, writing about the mistake, I just blame it on the high. In the high, I made a decision. Fucking, whatever. I'm going to run mile thirteen in under seven minutes. Mile twelve is 7:39.

I run about as hard as I can run, and don't show me the science; I know I'm moving fast. *Where's that 1:45 pace runner?* I think. *Did I blink and run right past them? All good, I'll catch the 1:40 guy. Or girl. Can girls run this fast? I doubt it.* Ugh, c'mon. Putting my interior monologue's absurd sexism aside, I do have a legitimate chance of breaking 1:45, and I want it. If I can break 1:45, I'll have a real shot at a sub-eight-minute pace for an entire half marathon, and for me, that would be an enormous accomplishment. There's less than eight hundred meters left, and I try to run harder. I try to lean around a turn and power through it, and that's when I get a whoopsie. A tiny cramp on the inside of my left thigh. I instinctively shorten my stride and slow down to almost a stop. I'm okay. I think. I'm moving again. I'm okay. I try to kick back up to speed and think I feel something in the right hamstring. I force a shorter, relaxed stride and give a long exhale to blow the anxieties out of my brain. It's okay. It's almost done now. Do your best. I round the corner to see the finish line. I see the 1:45 flag in front of me crossing that line. Then I cross the finish line.

Mile thirteen was 7:28.

I don't know how fast I ran the 0.1, but the science suggests it took longer than eleven seconds. I'll never run *only* thirteen miles again. Finish the 0.1. The 0.1 makes a difference.

And this is it, the part of the chapter where I try to explain it. That dumb, post-game question: *Dustin, can you describe to us what you're feeling right now?* Sure.

Well, my average pace was 8:02.

The chip time for my race says 1:45:11.

I almost ran faster sooner. I could have cramped worse sooner. I think I straddled the line well, and the end result is the fastest I've ever run that far. At thirty-six, I am better than I've ever been, but, I don't know, the stats don't tell the whole story, you know? I just have so much pride and gratitude for my body. I just want to thank God for the opportunity.

Readers won't be able to tell, but I affect a weird accent for my post-race interview. Blame Ricky Bobby. I wake up in the morning and piss excellence. Blame Johnny Moxon. The Mox. I mean, Dustin

Riedesel is only one man, you know?

Obviously, there's no post-race interview. They're handing out two hundred limited edition mugs to the top one hundred male and female finishers. I don't win a mug. There's no one I know at the finish line. No one drapes a medal on me. I'm handed a medal as I keep the crowd moving. I pick up a CLIF Bar, a banana, and a water bottle. I walk to the car alone. As I walk, I listen to "Konstantine" by Something Corporate because I've heard it a thousand times and it still makes my heart feel feelings. I'm emotionally drained and want it to still work. It works. Confirmation of life. It's a long walk back to the car, and the next song I play is "International Players Anthem" by UGK. This song has little to do with my life, but I just like hearing Andre 3000 sing "Keep your heart, three stacks. Keep your heart." And I like feeling like I've kept my heart. My heart is it. My body is it. And it feels like they've both forgiven me. Cancer, alcoholism, my life's myriad of failures. I could have lost it, but I went and got it.

Dear reader, do you understand what it is? What we're running towards when we go get it? I don't feel like I'm explaining it well.

I heard a story once, about a little boy asking his father how big God is. There was a plane flying overhead, and the father pointed to it and asked, "How big is that airplane?"

"It's tiny, Dad."

So the dad loads his kid into the car, and they drive to the airport, and they look at the airplanes on the runway. "How big are those airplanes?"

"Dad, they're huuuuge!"

The dad laughs. "That's what God's like, son. The *closer* you get to Him, the *bigger* He is."

I can't pinpoint the "it" in that God story for you. But right now, after this race, I've never felt closer to my body, and my mind is circling that God story. And I'm thinking about it as I'm getting closer to home. I'm not thinking about my shoes at all. They might as well be part of my feet. I get out of the car and put the medal around my own neck. I can't wait for Walter to see it. I can't wait for KT to ask me about it. But it's more than the medal. It's more than the race. The race would mean less to me without these specific people who rely on me and believe in me. And the truth I could've denied until now is that *they* would mean less to me without the race. Is it happiness? If so, it's different than I'm used to. I feel what must be an aspect of me but also feels like my grandpa, my dad, my brother. It's proud of me. Whatever it is, it is good. It is something I've worked hard to experience, and the work has increased my capacity to experience it. This is my reward. My post-race celebration will be telling KT. I won't explain any of it well, but my eyes will be shining, and I will be smiling, and for a beautiful time, it will all be so big and so close.

Weeks 17 & 18
The Long Runs

I wake up, and I do not piss excellence. That's me being transparent, unlike my urine. I like my urine to be clear-ish, but typically there's a very yellow tint. I assume there's nothing excellent about this. This is the kind of piss any Johnny-come-lately could produce. It's amateur piss, but now that I'm thinking about it, I feel good about amateur piss. Normal pee is a sign of a normal prostate, and I don't need an abnormal avocado of a prostate giving me irregular urine. I've run too far with this urine talk, but running far is what this book is about, and our male readers should know that getting over 3 hours a week of aerobic exercise dramatically decreases the risk of death via prostate cancer. Running: Take your prostate to a pro state.

Unrelated: If Nike ever needs some fresh copywriting ideas for their running division, I'm available. Like, really, totally available.

Anyway, I don't wake up and piss metaphorical excellence either. There's a saying that a lot of people have said, but somehow legendary Indiana basketball coach Bobby Knight gets prime credit. "Everyone wants to win, but not everyone wants to prepare to win." Even though I have absolutely zero chance of ever winning any race with more than ten participants, this quote applies to me. I love race day. My will to run well on race day is excellent. But waking up the week after a race and rediscovering the will to prepare for the next race? Well, I'm an amateur. I piss normal.

In week 17 of training for the Disney Marathon, I run forty-two miles with a long run of twenty-one miles. I post my training plan for the week on Instagram with a caption that reads, "I'm hugely encouraged by these past few months of training. When I first decided I wanted to do some distance running in 2018, I went all out on a treadmill to see what my best three miles was. It was twenty-nine minutes, a 9:40/mi pace. Now, I can run an eight-minute pace for thirteen miles. The meaning of the metrics isn't speed, but the self confidence that comes with sticking to something hard. Happy to be running." I must be tired. The only reason to write with that much motivational cheese is to convince myself that I'm *not* tired. But I *am* tired. I run seven miles on Monday. Seven miles on Tuesday. Five miles on Wednesday. Rest. Three miles on Friday.

Then it's long-run Saturday. I run a slow warm-up mile at a 10:30 pace. Then I kick up a little. I run the next fourteen miles at a 9:40 pace, which should be no big deal, but I'm battered. Maybe I messed up my nutrition, my hydration, I don't know. I bonk at mile fifteen, and I bonk hard. My legs are all cramping muscles and stiff tendons. I should stop, but the marathon is less than a month away. I tell myself that I *need* these miles. I tell myself that if I drop below a pace of fifteen minutes per mile that I'm done. I dig my heels in, and I'm being somewhat literal because the next hour is lived on my heels. I can't bend my legs well, and my calves are shot, so step after step is my entire weight being caught directly on my heel, impacting through my ankle and knee and hip with almost no support from the surrounding muscle groups. I imagine the force of the asphalt being relayed up the stack of joints like a triple combo of pool balls. This goes on for over an hour at a thirteen-minute-per-mile pace. It is a long time to struggle and, in retrospect, it was stupid. I finally quit at twenty miles. I'm broken. I can't do the last mile. I just can't.

This is the nadir of my marathon confidence. My body's electrolyte and carb needs are a complete mystery. There's no time left. The weeks of training have been a waste. All that body forgiveness from the Raleigh Half dries up with my sweat as I limp home. I am a failure.

In week 18 of training for the Disney marathon, I run forty-three miles with a long run of twenty-two miles. It's the last truly long run before I taper, and after last week, I'm scared. What if I bonk again? I guess I'll have to adjust my target pace to aim for a 4:20 Marathon? That would at least still be a PR. What if I don't even PR at Disney? I hear my train of thought and immediately switch the tracks. No need to route through Catastrophizing Grand Central. Besides, the run doesn't go *that* badly. I keep the pace slow the entire time, around ten minutes. Twenty-two miles in three hours and forty minutes. My body didn't break down with the time under tension. If I can endure that time at a higher pace, I can do it.

But can I do it? I don't really know. I choose to believe I can do it. I'm committed, so confidence is just a more comfortable emotion than doubt. Despite what signing up for a marathon implies, I prefer to be comfortable.

Recovery is progress. Oh no, is this a paradox? I'm glad you asked because the answer is yes.

And no.

Hey, it's a paradox—that's how it works.

If you are myopic, if your perspective is too tightly constricted to a particular race or run, then no, recovery is probably not progress. It's probably just recovery. However, if you step back and realize that the goal is to build a better runner and not just a better run, then recovery is obviously progress. Some people like the idea that the run is destruction and the recovery is what builds the runner back better than before. If that's your belief, fine. I don't subscribe. For me, it's all progress. Even the very moment I'm injured, it is progress. It's the most massive setback I can endure, but even writing that sentence tells you I'm enduring. I'm instantly sending emotional reinforcement. Physically, rehab will be progress too. What about a night of drinking that leaves me poisoned? Even then, I've plotted the first point in a story of forgiveness and resiliency. That's recovery. So it's progress. Just pull back farther. Make the perspective larger and more accepting.

In week 19 of training for the Disney Marathon, I run thirty-seven miles with a long run of sixteen miles. This is the beginning of a three-week taper. I run six 800m intervals at a 7:30 pace on Tuesday, but otherwise, all the miles are easy miles. Also, it's Christmas. My favorite holiday, especially since Walter and Winnie arrived. Seeing their excitement allows me to feel my own childhood again, when Christmas was still a miracle. Even as a kid, I never believed in Santa bringing me toys because I was quote-unquote "good." I knew I didn't deserve the tree full of presents. Christmas was truly a gift, and my parents taught me to be grateful. I want to teach my own kids to think less about what they deserve, to focus more on what they can earn, and no matter what, be grateful for the gifts they have. Then they'll be prepared for all of life's roads.

In week 20 of training for the Disney Marathon, I run thirty miles with a long run of twelve miles. New Year's Eve turns into New Year's Day. There have been hard days and failures, but when I pull back and think of the entire year, I'm grateful for the failures too. Nearly every night of the past year, I've rocked my son to sleep. He crawls onto my shoulder and says, "It was a good day." Then we say all the stuff he did that day. Not all the stuff inside the day is good, but the day is always good. No matter what happens at Disney, I know I can look at this past year's training and say with a full heart, "It was a good year."
And then it's here.

In week 21 of training for the Disney Marathon, I will run 35.2 miles, with a long run of 26.2 miles. I will run the Disney Marathon. Even now, writing these words months after the race itself, I am nervous. During week 21, the race is like my own death. It is one of those things I have to actively not think about or I start feeling unhelpful amounts of anxiety. But I can't not think about it, so I do what I do when I need to change the way my mind works. I jog my easy miles, and I start writing. I've already written a couple chapters of this book in week 21, but most of my writing is focused on my daughter. Her first birthday is the Thursday before the marathon. I write a birthday letter to my daughter, but because my art is undisciplined, the letter ends up being mostly about running.

In the "it doesn't get talked about enough" hall-of-fame movie, *Serendipity*, Jeremy Piven is an obituary writer who writes a letter to his friend. That letter is his friend's obituary, and Piven says, "Turns out I had writer's block and that's what ended up coming out. Blame it on the day job." I haven't seen or talked about that movie in a decade, but that line stuck with me. Maybe just for this very moment here. What would you call that?

When I realized my daughter's birthday letter was about running, I decided it should be the introduction to this book. However, as I was writing I realized the book was about something different than the letter, so the letter feels like it belongs here, with the emotions that birthed it. I won't put the whole thing here—it gets wordy, if you can imagine—but some condensed portions belong here.

Read those portions. After that, it's time to run a marathon.

Dear Winnie
A Letter To My Daughter on Her First Birthday

January 5th, 2022

January 5th, 2022

Dear Winnie,

Happy Birthday! You are one year old today!

This letter is also an introduction, and it's a rare introduction because I'm actually writing it before I've written the book. I intend to call the book *Looks Like We're Running*, and I think it's about choosing to do something even though it's painful and scary. So maybe it's about vulnerability and courage? I'm not one hundred percent sure yet. In the movie *Three Kings*, George Clooney says, " You do the thing you're scared shitless of, and you get the courage after you do it, not before you do it." Writing can be like that too. You write about the thing you're unsure of, and you get the clarity after you write it. That's why the introduction of a book is often the last thing written.

But life isn't a book. I can't flip to the last page and tell you how it's going to turn out. Instead, I can only share my experience. I hope there are times you'll see my experiences as a mirror, not because I want your life to look like mine, but because my greatest ambition as your father is to help you see yourself more clearly. Knowing yourself all the way through is one of life's greatest rewards, but it is also painful and scary.

In four days, I'll run the Disney Marathon. I've been wrestling with the meaning of it. How is running 26.2 miles like loving the entire life of my little girl? Don't expect a proof here. This isn't math, but sometimes a tangible experience helps me understand the effort necessary for larger abstractions, like how a contact lens bends the flood of light into a clear vision of the world. Running is a lens. Writing is a lens. Different prescriptions for my body and my mind, and if they're both dialed in, maybe I can see all the way through to the incomprehensible miracle inside my chest. That's where you are, Winnie. You give me feelings so big that I have to stretch the capacities of my lungs and metaphors to make room for the swells in my heart.

Before you showed up, I worried about having a girl. How would I relate to a girl? Could I teach her anything? Could I love her the right way? Silly concerns in hindsight because the person who showed up wasn't some blurry idea of a girl. It was you, and you were Winnie, and I have endless love for you.

A quick paragraph about love:

Life will force you to question love. What is it? Do you have it? Do others have it for you? Let me offer a dual-prescription on how to see love. It is one lens of hope and one lens of bravery. If you can look at a person, a situation, and especially yourself with hope for the outcome and bravery for the action, then love has prevailed and you can find your way forward. That is what The Beatles meant when they sang *All You Need is Love*. Love isn't an opiate. Love is a plan.

So, I'm running a marathon.

Hey, I didn't say love was a *good* plan. Sometimes you don't even like the plan, but disliking something does not make it automatically dismissable.

Your entire life, people will question your plans. For me, as a thirty-six-year-old, that questioning is usually stated, "What do you do?" But for the majority of my life, that question was, "What do you *want* to do?" Sometimes people would tack on "when you grow up" as if that's something people do. I never had a good answer, and it took me decades to realize that's the secret.

First off, who has answers at the beginnings of things? The first thirty years of life are mostly just a long series of introductions.

Secondly, a good answer to "what" is irrelevant. Plans should be less about what you do and more about who you do them for. And the most important person you need to explain that to is yourself. As the American philosopher Howard Thurman said, "Don't ask what the world needs. Ask what makes you come alive and go do it. Because what the world needs is people who have come alive." The secret to knowing what to do with your life is to never forget that it's *your* life. The plan is to love it well.

It turns out that I love running. I enjoy goaling an outcome slightly beyond my current ability. I enjoy overcoming the daily pain. I enjoy the joke I play on myself: Every time I hear a little voice inside of me say to take a day off, I say, "Maybe tomorrow," and I feel that little voice relax at the pleasant idea of a softer tomorrow, and it has no idea that tomorrow won't be a day off either. I enjoy achieving that outcome I nervously projected because I've created the fact that I am capable of more. Time and effort make me invincible. And yes, I even enjoy when I fail to achieve that slightly better outcome, because the little voice telling me to quit suddenly thinks it is big and powerful.

"Just quit. This is stupid," it says, and I feel an almost maniacal glee at how this worried piece of me doesn't know me at all.

"Maybe tomorrow," I say.

"You'll quit tomorrow?"

"No."

All this crazy inner dialogue is probably not uncommon for runners. The human brain is really just a comparison engine, and most runners' greatest rival is their past self. Cultivating an honest-to-God split personality would probably be beneficial to performance.

What's any of this have to do with you, Winnie? Well, I've thought a lot about running, but I'm also thinking about life, yours and mine. I'm going to compare life to a race. It's hacky. Seriously, everyone who's ever written has done this. Races are progress over time, uphills and downhills, competitors and solitude, and success is knowing you did your best. If life analogies were beer, races would be Bud Light, average and ubiquitous. That said, drink an ice-cold Bud Light at the first college football tailgate of the season. There's a time and place for everything.

This is only my second marathon. My goal is to run it under four hours. That's a meager pace for strong runners, but sub-four hours will be the toughest athletic accomplishment of my life. Should I fail, I'll try again. Should I succeed, I'll try to run an even faster time. The little voice inside me rages at the meaninglessness of it all, but the thing I understand that the voice does not is this: Good things require hard days, and the good thing is not the time. The time is merely evidence of the good thing, like a trophy memorializing the resilience beneath victory. The good thing is my own Peace of Mind.

Sub-four or not, I have Peace of Mind. I win it daily, moment by moment. I win it when I lace up the shoes. I win it by pushing intensity on a climb. I win it when my job is screaming to do it now, and I calmly let the job know it will be done after I run. Winnie, whenever you encounter life's burdens of various size, if you can pick them up *voluntarily*, then they will cease to be burdens at all, and you will carry them with Peace of Mind.

But also, Peace of Mind is won when I give myself a day to recover. It's won by decreasing pace in extreme heat. It's won when, the moment after I've laced up my shoes, my wife asks if I want to take the kids to the park, and I untie my shoes because running can wait. Winnie, maybe it won't be running for you, but it will be something. Never forget, you *chose* to pick it up, and if it becomes burdensome, you can set it down. It will be there waiting for you when you're ready.

Don't confuse Peace of Mind with Zen or tranquility. Running is a fucking war, and battles leave you crying with pain and laughing with joy. It's in those extreme states, when you've pushed yourself so hard that you can't find comfort in any crevice of your own body, that you get to learn something important about your own mind. For me, it's this: It's *my* mind. No one made me run far and hard. No one inflicted this pain upon me. Maybe I didn't ask to exist, but I have a life all the same, and I chose to run with it. This is *my* pain and *my* joy. I will fight for them and hope for more. Because joy and pain can't be divided. They are halves of the same, complete beauty. When you experience that beauty, you see yourself differently than before. Pain comes from the fight. Joy comes from hope fulfilled. Some people fear that pain comes from hope unfulfilled, but they're not correct. Hope unfulfilled is depression, and depression can only take hold when you are no longer willing to fight. To fight *is* to hope.

Then what of fulfillment? What of joy? Am I simply destined to fight forever? Yes, hahaha! That is exactly my plan! Even if I run a sub-four-hour time at Disney, I will compare someone's sub-three-hour pace to my shuffle and think, "*They* look like a *runner*." And then I will smile and wish them as much hope and joy as I have found. Winnie, my fulfillment is *you*. I hoped for you to be born and I was fulfilled. I hoped to see you smile and I was fulfilled. I hoped to see you walk and get up after you fell, and I was fulfilled. The joy of my life is that I don't know who you're going to be, and yet I get to see you become exactly who you are. I'm not just a dad. I'm *your* dad, and loving the entirety of *your* life will be the highlight of mine.

The race is long, and the only thing that matters is that I run it well. I'm scared. I'm excited, too. That's perfect. I have hope and bravery, and there's no way I'd rather live.

For all the many times in your life when you feel confused about your place in the world, never ignore the clarity of purpose you gave to the man who wrote these words. Because of you, he ran to the best of his ability. He was certain of why he chose his direction, and he was delighted by the struggle and reward in every step he took.

Week 21
The Disney Marathon

Have you spent this entire book wondering why KT and I chose Disney over some other marathon? No? Well, I'm telling you anyway. We live in Raleigh. Disney is in Orlando. Halfway between is Bluffton, South Carolina. KT's brother Ben and his wife Kira live in Bluffton. When KT and I were sitting in that Florida beach house with twenty other family members considering a marathon, we mentioned the Disney race was in January. Kira said she'd be happy to watch the kids that week. Nowhere to be seen, Ben agreed. That's why we chose Disney. If someone could watch the kids for race day, everything else about the training was just details. I gave The Mouse our money.

Now we're driving to The Mouse. It's our first weekend away from the kids in sixteen months. You'd think we'd just want a hotel room, a warm bath, and some candles, maybe turn on the Sisqo CD, see what happens. But no, we're driving to a marathon. Where's the romance, you ask? Let me explain. Our first stop is at a Parker's gas station exactly 0.6 miles from where KT and I have left our kids. We couldn't wait. One of the true joys of having kids is realizing how awesome everyday life really is. You realize that mundane activities have always been infused with a deep, tranquil Zen that allows you to experience the beauty inherent to all of God's creation. Absent the kids, we can bathe in that mundane Zen. Two hearts, exhausted but transcendent; this is its own kind of romance. Plus, this Parker's gas station has a lot going for it. The bathroom doesn't make you ask for a key, and the attendant always reports your bill due in pennies. "Coffees will cost 432 pennies." Absurd. One day, I'm actually gonna stop in at that Parker's with a—I don't know—a shaving bag of pennies and just thunk it down in front of this guy. *Who's amusing themselves now, Chuckles? You count the pennies.* Have I lost the Zen-slash-romance in this stop? How about this: Parker's has a great coffee bar. There are enough varieties of International Delight creamer to make the first seven times feel like the first time. I counted. There are seven flavors of creamer. All that variety and I bust a hazelnut! I'm a man. Easy to please. For KT, I get her a cream collaboration between International Delight and Hershey's. Yeah, *that* Hershey's. The wrapper that looks like what's on the inside. Chocolate is the currency of affection, and this creamer is Hershey's Chocolate Caramel. Does the caramel add more or less affection? I don't know. I don't overthink it. I also get us a big bottle of water to split like Lady and The Tramp. So yeah, the romance is alive.

The race is tomorrow morning and I haven't run in three days. We stop at a gas station in Jacksonville. It's no Parker's, but it sits beside a school and a low-traffic suburb. KT and I jog two "shake-out" miles. I feel bouncy. I feel strong. We cruise two miles at a 9:40 pace and my heart rate never peaks above 120 beats per minute. KT is also delighted at how good she feels. Did the taper really work? Could we actually be ready for this marathon?

We arrive in Orlando and head to the race expo at the ESPN Wide World of Sports Complex. The complex is huge and amazing, but the expo is not great. For the uninformed, an expo is where you pick up your race bib and t-shirt. Expos are typically built like a labyrinth to slide a worming crowd over the hooks of every vendor fishing for money from the running public. I usually find such bald-faced capitalism endearing, but this expo is tired. It has been running for four days. Disney's marathon weekend starts on Thursday with a 5K and escalates to a 10K on Friday, a half marathon on Saturday, and the Marathon on Sunday. This allows all runs to happen early, before the parks open, and it allows runners to run multiple races. Multiple races? Yeah, people do it. The Goofy Challenge is running both the half and full marathons, and this earns a special medal. The Dopey Challenge runs all four races, 5K to full marathon, and not only earns a Dopey Challenge medal, but also the Goofy Challenge medal. The people doing these challenges are insane in an admirable way, and if we attended this expo on Wednesday with that crowd, I'm sure it would be a hive of batshit energy. But it's Saturday. This expo wants to break down. The t-shirts are picked over. Booth workers are trying to avoid eye contact as much as we are. However, we leave on a grace note. The Athletic Brewing booth was overstocked. Take a beer. Take two. They don't want to carry it back. Athletic Brewing makes my favorite non-alcoholic beers. We stock up. It will taste great in a hotel shower after running 26.2 miles.

Our hotel is the Wilderness Lodge. I'm not actually sure if I'm ethically out of bounds to call it the Wilderness Lodge versus *Disney's* Wilderness Lodge. I'm not worried about Disney taking legal action, but I'd hate to offend more generic lodges in actual wilderness, so we'll keep the tag. Disney's Wilderness Lodge is huge and immaculate. The lobby ceiling is one hundred feet high atop stone and timber. KT mentions how abnormally clean it is. The place is full, restaurants booked and lobby seating occupied, but I don't see janitors bustling around. Maybe the feather dusters and mops just work themselves around here. Do you believe in magic? We check in. The kid behind the desk is likely an aspiring actor, and he's playing the role of Hospitality Worker 1 so well that I feel genuine gratitude. I ask if there's access to a microwave so I can make oatmeal at 2:00 a.m. before the race. He says there's no public microwave, but they'll have a microwave brought to my room within the hour. He turns and winks a telepathic request, and Hospitality Worker 2 clicks her heels and flies off to find a microwave. I'm deep into my mid-thirties, and I get Disney World.

This place is great.

Then KT and I are sitting on a dock, overlooking the Bay Lake on which a ferry will carry us to the Magic Kingdom. We have dinner reservations at 3:30 in the afternoon. With any luck, we will be in bed by seven, getting as much sleep as possible for a race that begins at five o'clock in the morning. We talk about how nice it is to be alone before immediately talking about bringing the kids. I want to borrow their eyes. They would see the magic of a real-life boy and none of the puppeteer's strings. Without them, we squint, and it's pretty close. We see characters we've known since childhood parade down Main Street into Cinderella's castle. We eat pad Thai at the Jungle Cruise Cantina. We hold big ice cream cones as we saunter back to the ferry.

The presentation of it all is so impressive, and while I prepare my clothes and food for the morning, I mentally adjust my idea of Disney. I used to think condescendingly of Disney as a surface merchant. They simply took regular things like dinner and ice cream and festooned them to a degree so unrecognizable that they could call it an elevated experience and charge you three months of mortgage. Now, it is hard work to be an elevated thing. It takes intention, endurance and strength. Whether or not Disney truly *is* an elevated experience or not, that's a matter of personal perspective. But what I know for sure is this: Disney wishes to be an elevated experience. And it is also hard work to *look* like the thing you wish to be. My idea of Disney hasn't fundamentally changed, but I remove the condescension. Disney is grinding. I respect that.

I sleep easily. The 2:00 a.m. alarm should feel terrible, but the pre-race energy skews my reality. Oatmeal, peanut butter, two bananas, coffee, and water are all consumed. My only concern is that I don't have to poop. I badly want to poop, not because I'm constipated or feel the physical need to poop, but because pooping would allow me to relax, to know that every pre-race box is checked.

Unfortunately, my body is not scheduled to poop before 3:00 a.m., so it doesn't happen

In case you're debating whether you would like to run the Disney Marathon, put this comment in the "pros" column. The trains run on time. KT and I simply woke up, walked to the front of our hotel, and got on the bus. We sat with others in a collective sense of nerves and optimism for about forty minutes before being dropped directly where we needed to be. No parking, no navigation, no additional stress. The race started at the Experimental Prototype Community of Tomorrow. Some folks call it EPCOT. The bag check was fast and conveniently located, and the lines to the portapotties were incredibly short because there were so many damn portapotties. If you haven't run many races, it's hard to emphasize how grateful one feels for an abundance of portapotties.

I still haven't pooped. Start time is seventy-five minutes away. I make a gut call. I have a second coffee. I also buy and drink another water, thinking it will keep my hydration balanced. Does the coffee work? I don't want to soil coffee's good name just because I couldn't soil a toilet. I do squeeze out a tiny nugget before heading to the starting line, so sure, it worked.

We walk beside thousands to the starting line. Some look like real runners. Some don't, but they're all here. Ninety percent of running is just showing up. A lot of people look like Disney characters. Tutus, pixie wings, and running gear that resembles Disney Princess outfits are all common. One guy near me and KT is dressed so authentically as Captain Jack Sparrow that only logical probability keeps me from believing he is Johnny Depp. While it looks as if he built the boots around running shoes, he is still running in full pants, knee-length jacket, dreadlocked wig, pirate hat, and, as if that isn't enough, he has a holstered sword clanging against his leg with every step. That's a lot of baggage for 26.2 miles. I look at him, and I don't savvy. Like, at all. The only justification for running in such an outfit is so you can stand at the starting line, and just before the starting fireworks, you look at the people around you and say, "This is the day you will always remember as the day you almost caught Captain Jack Sparrow." Even so, that whole outfit is a heat trap.

And it's already hot enough. We hoped for a forty-five-degree start, but it is sixty-three degrees at 5:00 a.m. It will be in the mid-seventies by sunrise. I'm worried that my fuel and hydration plan will turn to ashes in this heat. I have four gels, and there are Powerade aid stations every two miles. I did the math, one gel every forty-five minutes and six ounces of Powerade every two miles should equate to 60g of carbs per hour. Just to be safe, I will eat all the chews, bananas, and candy bars at select aid stations. I am uncertain about my hydration needs, but the Powerade and gels should get me right next to 700mg of sodium per hour, which lands in the recommended range. I tell myself that heat only makes it hot. I tell myself the gameplan is still sound.

We're at the starting line. KT and I both get nervous and leave the corral for a last-minute pee break. She runs to a portapotty. I hop the barrier and use the woods. We rush back, afraid of missing the gun, then wait for another twenty minutes as other corrals are released. I look for the four-hour pace flag, but never see one. I tell myself I'm trained. I'll run my own race. It will be fine.

Our corral is released. KT and I kiss or fist bump or something, and then I create some space. We could run a couple miles together, but I think we both prefer to get away from the pressure of another person's pace. KT says she just wants to finish, but she's made a lot of jokes about Oprah running 4:29. It's funny, but I don't think it's a joke. She's trying to beat Oprah.

I'm trying to beat four hours, and I have no idea what's going to happen.

If you look at my splits, the first two miles look relaxed and measured. But what something looks like and what it really is are two different things. This race is twenty thousand people jammed shoulder to shoulder with no uniformity of pace. Runners are passing walkers falling behind joggers dodging stopped stretchers. I'm wary of this phase of the race. I ran over twenty-seven miles to complete my last marathon because I ran a serpentine path to navigate the crowded road. This time, I jog slow, waiting for a path to open up where I can increase my speed. My anxiety builds with my twelve-minute-per-mile pace until a curve in the road or a break in the crowd, and then I release pressure with a twenty-second, high-pace burst before getting bottled up. The other option is to get off the road and run in the grass beside the road, but it's still dark. The only light comes intermittently from streetlights. Without being able to see the terrain, I'm fearful of a sprained ankle. But others are on the grass. They pass me on my left like I'm The Falcon and they're Captain America. I risk it. The grass is tougher than the road, but the sense of claustrophobia is lessened. Despite the herky-jerky start, Mile one is 9:01. Good. I relax. Mile two is 9:29.

Seeing nine and a half minutes freaks me out. I'm off pace. I get back on the roads. I'm back to the sporadic speed. I chill when I'm bottled up, and when I have an opening, I stride out and make up the difference. This may be bad strategy, but it feels great. I feel way better than either half, and those races ended with speed. The taper most certainly worked. My legs are strong, all I need to do now is trust them. Mile three is 8:33.

I've found my first kindred spirit in the race. He's a big guy, well-muscled. His shirt is army green, so I ascribe some militaristic bullheadedness to him. He and I have been passing each other since the starting line. While I speed up and slow down to maintain a shortest path from turn to turn, he weaves around people who are going too slow. He accepts no retreat in his pace. That's *so* army guy. I respect the drive. I also run my openings harder to keep up. Mile four is 8:26.

Just like 9:29 freaked me out, seeing 8:26 also freaks me out. I'm running hot, and I know I need to slow down. But I feel great, and I'm still running slower than either of my half times. Maybe I'm not running hot. Maybe I'm running exactly as fast as I should be running. Maybe the only problem with my pace is that I'm burning too many brain calories thinking about my damn pace. The crowd is finally stringing out. The course pours onto some open lanes of blocked off highway. There's an aid station here, and all the volunteers are wearing purple shirts with the Leukemia & Lymphoma Society logo on the front. That's pretty cool. I grab two cups of Powerade, walking to drink them steadily. I also grab a water to balance the thickness of my first gel. I have no idea if you need water to balance a gel, but it's something I've done in the past so I'm doing it now. Mile five is 8:41.

In a perfect world, I'd get to twenty miles around the three-hour mark, running nine-minute miles. And in this perfect world, I'd have plenty of juice left to dial it up to 8:30 miles, finishing just a few minutes under the four-hour mark to beat my previous best by twenty-five minutes. Will I be able to run harder in the last six than I ran in the previous twenty? It seems audacious, but not impossible. I just ran a few 8:30-ish miles and they felt like no effort at all. Plus, there's going to be so much emotion to tap into for the finish. Andrea Hunter Cadavid is a friend. She gave me a tip. Paraphrasing, she said, "When I run a marathon, I write the six names on my arm of people who mean the most to me, and I dedicate each of the last six miles to one of those people. You'll run that one mile for that one person very hard. And the next mile for the next person. You won't give up on them. Your body can take it. You just have to believe in your body." Now, Andrea's marathon PR is 2:47:19, so she is legitimately elite. Maybe what works for her won't work for me, but damnit it sounds good. I have six people I care about. I can dig deep. Mile six is 8:59.

I'm so lost in my own race that Disney's schtick hasn't registered with me. I run right by the frequent options to stop and take photos with characters. Some of these characters are only found in this race, and this is big for the Disney diehards. Me? I'm not stopping unless I see Dwayne "The Rock" Johnson himself posing in full Skipper Frank Wolff regalia. Spoiler alert—and this spoiler is for this book, not the pseudo-historical fantasy quest that is Disney's *Jungle Cruise*—The Rock does not make an appearance. Beyond the character photos, we've only run through EPCOT. It was less than a mile of the six. We're on Florida highway for at least another two miles until Magic Kingdom. Mile seven is 8:50.

The highway portion of running Disney is easily the worst part. It's not boredom. I've never been bored during a race. Actually, I don't think I've been bored in the last three years. Through the proper combination of writerly curiosity, job busyness, toddler fatigue, and runner's Zen, I'm never bored. However, I am occasionally annoyed. And that's the issue with this highway. We spend lengthy bits of course heading up and down looping exit ramps slanted to accommodate cars traveling over thirty-five miles per hour. Check my math, but that's a forty-five-minute marathon time, and I'm not running that fast. The road is too slanted for my pace, and this is exacerbated by the fact that one of my legs is slightly shorter than the other. I mostly ignore this imbalance in my life, but now it is the single most annoying fact of my body. For the first time in these 26.2 miles, I think that I am probably not built for this. At least I outlasted my self-doubt for roughly the first third of the race. Props to training. Mile eight is 8:54.

The solely physical portion of the race is over. I start noticing twitches in my legs and pulses in my feet. My body is talking to me, engaging my intellect to stop the madness. I don't fight it. I just talk back. *Hey Dust, you're doing good. You know for a fact you'll hold up for the next hour. Slower than the half means longer than the half. You're right on time.* I run down a hill and under a bridge. As I come back up, there is a huge, roadside booth representing the Leukemia & Lymphoma Society. They're cheering. They have no way of knowing I'm a survivor, but I point to them and yell, "LET'S GO!" Mile nine is 8:51.

The bright side of starting a January race at 5:00 a.m. is that I'm running my tenth mile of the morning and it's still dark out. It's also muggy. My light green tank top is now just a green tank top, and my hat has absorbed sweat to the very end of it's short, flat bill. My mind is hyper alert to discomfort because my body is beginning to pester my brain. "We've been running long enough." That voice is loud. I haven't heard the music in my headphones for five straight songs. It would take world-class entertainment to distract me now. Mile ten is 8:56.

Coming through a tunnel, I hear cowbells and clapping. I know as it is happening that this is a moment that I won't ever forget. I emerge from the tunnel to turn directly onto Main Street of the Magic Kingdom. The shops and buildings are lit up. The streets are crowded with people cheering for the runners. And at the end of the road is Cinderella's castle, sparkling and lighting up the night sky like it has lit my TV screen before a hundred childhood stories. The spectacle gives me goosebumps, and I don't fight my smile as the castle grows. I run in and through the castle and imagine myself watching a Disney movie with Walter and Winnie and telling them that Dada's been there, that it's a real place. That will be cool. Mile eleven is 8:53.

I have pacers! It was so natural. This lovely couple was running just the right speed, and now my pace is perfect with zero thought whatsoever. I just follow along. The guy is a runner. It's obvious. He has powerful legs and a bird-bone upper body. He carries no gear except his watch. His gate is fluid and easy. The girl is fit, but she's working harder than he is. Their outfits explain their effort. She wears a hydration pack. She's dressed like the Queen of Hearts, with capri tights that are red on one leg and black on the other and a top that flips the colors. There's a crown and playing card icons, all well-assembled. The guy is wearing black shorts and a red shirt.

Together, it all works, like a Queen and a Jack completing a straight. A solid, well-paced straight. Miles twelve and thirteen are 8:43 and 8:42.

My half marathon split is one hour and fifty-six minutes. That's good. My plan is to follow the Queen and Jack as long as they can keep it up. The only time we break ranks is aid stations. They walk every aid station, so I run ahead, get my Powerade, and then start walking myself. I wait for them to run past me before picking up pace behind them. I have no idea if they're aware of me, but if they are, they don't seem to care. They stop to pee, and so do I. The portapotties are open, and I'm quick, paranoid that I'll lose them. I don't. I emerge. They emerge. They run. I follow. Mile fourteen is 8:45.

It's funny how the mind works. When I'm running five miles, the fourth mile feels like a monster. When you run twenty-six miles, the fourteenth mile feels casual. I've been running for two hours, and it might as well have been twenty minutes. Then, I feel a "whoopsie" in my right hamstring. My face spasms as fear scratches the back of my eyelids. *Not cramps. Not this early.* I walk. I rally my focus. I jog. *Easy on the kick back.* I watch the Queen and Jack fading forward, and I pick up the pace. The same hamstring spasms again, so I slow down. *Okay. Relax. Shorter strides.* I walk through the next aid station. I stretch out to touch my toes. I slam four Powerades. I take my third gel. Mile fifteen is 9:26.

The triage at the aid station seems to work. Movement is cautious but steady. Upping the Powerade intake will work. It has to. I'm back on track. Mile sixteen is 8:53.

I'm trying to solve the last ten miles as I run. Is this fuel or is this hydration? Does it matter? Bonking, cramping, hitting the wall. I've listened to hours of podcasts on this very topic. Running Explained. The Marathon Training Academy. The Strength Running Podcast. The Bare Performance Podcast. They all agree. Once the cramping has started mid-race, it's too late to catch up. I also hear a little voice inside of me, and I realize it's not the usual one goading me to quit. The voice might actually be *me*, admitting that I never understood hydration. I crammed some info about electrolytes after that terrible twenty-mile run in week 17, but I never really incorporated it. At some point, another whoopsie. My form is already compromised, but I adjust further. I hammer more Powerades. I panic drink water because I don't know what I need. Chews, bananas, whatever I can find. I can be slow for a couple miles if it saves my body from complete shutdown. Mile seventeen is 9:26. Mile eighteen is 9:47.

Not unlike Chicago, I have a brief moment of fortune. This is the one moment of the race where KT and I pass each other. I'm leaving the Animal Kingdom as KT's entering it. She yells my name and I pick my head up from the ground and instinctively smile. I think I threw her the Shaka, a Hawaiian gesture for "Things are great." Whatever. KT knows I'm from Kansas. Seeing me say "Hakuna Matata" with island gestures should have tipped her to my struggle, but she saw it differently. "You looked like you were doing great," she said. My confidence died a few miles back, and seeing KT was the last glimmer of hope. Mile nineteen is 9:59.

Watching my race fall apart in real time is an odd sensation. I've dreamed of seeing a PR time that flips the leftmost digit from a "4" to a "3," but for the last three miles, I've seen my average pace slow one second at a time. I look at it now, and it reads 8:59. Then, as I stare at it, I see the leftmost digit flip from an "8" to a "9." Mile twenty is 10:25.

"Okay, what am I doing here?"

The existential self-pity rolls in like a wave. I mean, I have freedom, and this is how I choose to live? My twenty-mile split is barely over three hours, and this is where I should think of my six people. But at this point, what's the point? But now I can't not think about my six people. I try to focus on one, but instead I get a silly, family fantasy montage. My brothers, sister, wife, and kids all welled up with pride as I grind relentlessly against long odds delivered on waves of pain. I am deep into the emotional portion of the race, and I'm bordering on tears as I limp and shuffle and imagine Walter talking about me as if I'm Superman. I'm such a piece of shit. Mile twenty-one is 11:11.

But what am I doing *here*?

My blood feels like battery acid. I imagine Tyler Durden giving me a chemical burn and telling me I'm experiencing premature enlightenment. *Stay present.* The sun rose forty-five minutes ago, and I'm now running directly towards it's taunting heat and unyielding glare. EPCOT, here I come. The stiff grimace in my face matches the rigid muscles of my body's salt-depleted body. There are Disney workers handing out towels soaked in ice water. I use it on my palms and neck. I wipe my face and realize where all my body's salt went as the sponge drags the granules across my forehead. It barely helps, but it passes some time. *Congratulations, you're one step closer to hitting bottom.* Mile twenty-two is 11:04.

What am I *doing* here?

I hear a big booming voice yell, "Green Shirt, I see you working! Keep going, big fella!" It's a DJ, and just being recognized puts some pep back into my step. I don't know why he called me out individually. I see a Biofreeze table. Biofreeze is a menthol pain gel that provides relief to sore muscles and joints. I normally think it's kind of a hoax, but I'm desperate. I stop and slather it on. The workers at the Biofreeze desk are looking at me like I'm a literal train wreck, and I realize why the DJ called me out as soon as they ask, "Do you want some vaseline?" My green shirt has two massive pepperonis of blood right over my nipples. I've never had the bloody nipple problem before, but this is a full-blown case. The workers hand me a towel to wipe the bio freeze off my hands. Scoops of Vaseline slather my nipples. I ramble gratitude and hobble on, grabbing Powerade and some sports jelly beans. It's a good stop. I'm surviving! Mile twenty-three is 11:00.

What am *I* doing here?

I'm failing. This is the official moment. My race has been steadily getting worse for one hour and thirteen minutes, but this is the moment I fully acknowledge my failure to run a sub-four-hour marathon. Even if I were magically restored and one hundred percent fresh, I couldn't run the remaining 5K in under twenty minutes. I let self-pity wash over me. I'm in terrible pain. Cramps have spread from my hamstrings to my quads and calves. Even my forearms are fighting cramps from holding the bent elbow for arm pumping. I smash my wooden legs into my rusty ankles. The front half of my foot refuses to receive any of my body weight, so my heels are basically peg legs slamming against concrete as I fall forward. Mile twenty-four is 11:11.

What am I doing here?

I'm improving. The acceptance of failure is almost simultaneous with the realization of success. My secondary goal is to run the fastest marathon of my life, and as long as my body does not completely shut down, I can do it. I ran 4:23 in Chicago. Can I get under 4:10 today? I do some math. It's possible. It's too soon to know what my reasons are for running this race, but maybe this will be one takeaway: I should have recognized the improvement sooner. The optimism is energy. This will be the fastest marathon of my life. Time to dump the self-pity and run like it. Mile twenty-five is 10:45.

Hilariously, I think, a big guy has caught up to me. It's Army Guy from the beginning of the race, only he's not looking militaristic anymore. He's obviously fighting cramps too. Hobbling as best he can. We trade leads a few times as hills and efforts wax and wane. We're both too tired to acknowledge any competition. Actually, there is no competition left. We're just dragging our bodies along, but I'm glad he's here. I can feel myself trying harder because of this stranger suffering like I am. Given that he and I are starting and ending together, I imagine his last hour has been a lot like mine, walking and slogging his way through the pain. But now, in one last push, it looks like we're running again, and breaking ten minutes is a triumph. Mile twenty-six is 9:53.

These final miles have been filled with fanfare; people are cheering and holding signs. I should be too tired to care, but I'm not. I do care. I'm grateful. I'm so ready to finish this race, and I'm grateful that these people want me to be finished too. The finish line has stands of people, music, and the giant, beautiful word "FINISH" on a tall banner. I run underneath it and my race is over. I take a medal. I stop at a table for a Powerade, a water, a banana, a snack box. I get out of the flow of traffic and take my shirt off. I dab the blood off my chest, put my medal on, and sip my Powerade as I limp through the winding barriers to the finisher's zone. Once there, I pick up my bag from gear check and wait for KT.

I want to sit down, but I am legitimately afraid that if I sit down, I will not be able to stand up. I just wait there, honestly disappointed in myself. Fortunately, I'm not waiting long. KT emerges. I'm waving my arms, and she's looking straight through me for five seconds before I see recognition dawn on her face. She smiles. I smile. We high five.

"Did you do it?" She asks.

I shake my head. "PR though, so that's good."

"Dust, that's awesome!" She says, and she sounds so genuinely proud of me that I believe it. It will take time to heal my wounded pride, but this compliment from my wife is the first band-aid. With her, I know that I will be proud of myself, and it reminds me of why I fell in love with her in the first place.

I ask KT how she did. She smiles. "Oprah can suck it!"

Official times are 4:11:57 for me and 4:28:15 for KT. I'm incredibly proud of her. She *does* turn thirty-five this year, and she's still got *it*. I have a suspicion that one day—much older than thirty-five—if we try to think back on when we were at our best, it will be hard to deny this phase of life. We have two young children, demanding jobs, friendships we work at, and we just finished our first and second marathons. This exhaustion is a choice, and I proudly say it was well-chosen. We look like old people walking with a slow, painful shuffle across the parking lot in search of our bus. But we hold hands with intention, endurance, and emotional strength. We look like we're happy. Maybe others don't see us that way, but that's just a matter of perspective. If you find yourself on the far side of a marathon finish line, squint a little. I hope you see what I see. It's a beautiful snapshot of life.

Weeks *Ad Infinitum*
The Answers at the Finish Line

Well, I failed. I did not run the Disney marathon in under four hours. It kind of makes for a bummer ending to a book. More frustratingly, the reasons I ran—the ones I thought I would become aware of after running the marathon—are not what I'd hoped they'd be. Five months of training to shave twelve minutes off a distance of 26.2 miles, and I actually have very little new information. I feel like I've been chiseling away at a rock day after day, curious about what's inside—it turns out, more rock.

Oh, sweet revelation. If only I were faster, perhaps I could catch you and make you mine. Or, maybe, I'll just sit here and bang my head against the rock some more.

Here's something I read about running, from my favorite book about running, Haruki Murakami's *What I Talk About When I Talk About Running*. Murakami is an extremely creative writer, a novelist, but this is a memoir, so in it, he talks a lot about his mental process. In doing so, Murakami shares an article he once read. In that article, a runner shares something his older brother told him about running. The older brother says, "Pain is inevitable. Suffering is optional." The runner ponders that phrase endlessly. After reading the article, so does Murakami. After reading Murakami, so do I. And now, with any luck, so will you.

I do not have to run the marathon. I own a Peloton Bike and a well-equipped home gym, and I understand the benefits of staying fit by other means. My body looks better when I'm lifting. I am more entertained when I am on the Peloton. I experience more community at 12th State Crossfit. And yet ... I'm still pondering the phrase, "Suffering is optional." I used to think the phrase was about positivity, that despite experiencing pain, I could choose to not add suffering to the pain with catastrophizing and agonizing. But as I ponder the option, I'm not sure it's about positivity. Compared to the relative joy of Crossfit, bodybuilding, and Peloton, the marathon is suffering. It is also optional. Perhaps that's exactly why I choose it.

KT and I joke about this book. For months, she was the only other person who had read any of it.

"Who's your audience?" She asks.

"The literate," I say.

"Readers!"

"It is designed *specifically* for that crowd."

"English only?"

"Too niche?"

"You might want an audio version."

And so it goes.

I chose the title *Looks Like We're Running* because I'm insecure about my running and my writing, and to me, this title said, "Hey, take it easy on me. I'm just an amateur." At some point during the training, I realized that amateurism is the point. Marriage, parenting, faith, friendship, running or any kind of exercise: rarely does one get paid for the most important aspects of their life, and hell, you can't take the money with you anyway. Life is an amateur event. David Foster Wallace once wrote, "The horrific struggle to establish a human self results in a self whose humanity is inseparable from that horrific struggle. That our endless and impossible journey toward home is in fact our home." You don't have to agree with this Wallace quote or run marathons to understand why people choose to do hard things. The suffering is optional. The choice is intentional. This is the amateur's mindset. You run to become a runner, and for doing so, you're given the lifetime achievement award of getting to run. So right now, for me, it looks like I'm running, but for you, the running can be writing or bowhunting or taxidermy or whatever because it's all the endless and impossible journey toward knowing yourself. As far as I can tell, the secret is this: The burden of suffering, voluntarily chosen, ceases to be suffering at all; the suffering becomes daily nourishment, and the only burden left is that you must feed yourself every day.

My favorite encapsulation of this point is from Philosopher Albert Camus. He wrestled constantly with how one should handle the chaotic and random trials life gives us by using the story of Sisyphus. Sisyphus was a king who tricked the gods, and as comeuppance, the gods assigned him to an eternity of rolling a boulder up a hill without ever reaching the top. Camus simply reimagined the punishment into reward. He said, "One must imagine Sisyphus happy."

And when I try to explain why imagining the experience of endlessly rolling a boulder up a hill can be anything but miserable, I share something Mark Manson wrote in *The Subtle Art of Not Giving a F*ck*: "The desire for a more positive experience is itself a negative experience. And, paradoxically, the acceptance of one's negative experience is itself a positive experience."

I've been fired, dumped, and ignored. I know what it feels like to be dropped off at rehab. I've been on my knees in a jail cell. I've laid awake in an ICU afraid that falling asleep might also mean not waking up. I've apologized. I've sobered up. I've accepted Christ. I've survived cancer. I'm thirty-six years old, but I've had a lot of experience in feeling bad and then feeling better. If anyone were to approach me directly for help in turning their life around, I think there's one thing I would do for them before anything else. I would smile as warmly as I can, hand them a pair of Nike's, and say, "Let's get you back on your feet."

You see, it doesn't matter what specifically is difficult in your life.

Life is generally difficult. To positively embrace its challenges requires not just choice, but intentional choice done repetitively. Life is a practice. Life is training. To understand this on any level is to understand it on every level. I've never read *The Book of Five Rings*, but I've heard Joe Rogan quote it a hundred times: "Know the Way broadly, and you will see it in all things." I know the way to train my body for a difficult day in the future, a day of accountability, and I work every day so that I will be up to the moment. Now, I see the way in being a father, a husband, a leader, an employee, a friend, and writer who wishes to see himself more clearly. I will pick up these burdens voluntarily, and I will train. Certainly, I will fail as much as I succeed, and maybe I will quit picking up the burdens one day. But not today. And not tomorrow either. I like picking up the burdens.

Imagine Sisyphus happy.

Haruki Murakami wrote *What I Talk About When I Talk About Running* after nearly twenty-five years of consistent running, including several marathons. He writes:

Any time I run a marathon, my mind goes through the same exact process. Up to nineteen miles, I'm sure I can run a good time, but past twenty-two miles, I run out of fuel and start to get upset at everything, and at the end, I start to feel like a car that's run out of gas. But after I've finished, and some time has passed, I forget all the pain and misery and am already planning how I can run an even better time in the next race. The funny thing is, no matter how much experience I have under my belt, no matter how old I get, it's all just a repeat of what came before. **I think certain types of processes don't allow for any variation. If you have to be part of that process, all you can do is transform--or perhaps distort-- yourself through that persistent repetition, and make that process a part of your own personality.**

You could argue that I don't have to be a part this marathon process. You're technically correct. I also don't have to have write or be married or show up for my kids. It's running, not death and taxes. But I'm probably too far down the road for that argument. Once the process that doesn't allow for variation has become a part of your own personality, then part of your personality doesn't allow for variation. The gods have given you your boulder.

In week one of training for the San Antonio Marathon, I run twenty-five miles with a long run of eight miles. My older brother and I are going to run San Antonio together. He ran the Austin Marathon a month after I ran Disney. Like me, he had designs to run under four hours, and like me, he missed it, though he fared better on a tougher course, running 4:04. We both cramped, ending our races in shuffling pain and walking-dead miles. We're both a little salty about it, and that's why we're going to run it again, damnit. At least, that's the reason I'm telling people who ask. Really, I'm not aware of the exact reasons why I'm running, but once I've finished *this* marathon, I'll understand exactly why I ran it.

The truth is just one more finish line away.

Acknowledgements

In general, people spend too little time in gratitude to those who helped them along the way. I will continue that rich tradition with a brief page. I swear it is sincere.

Thank you to my wife for teaching me conditional love. Conditional love is not an endless trust fund. It has to show up for work every day. It has to sacrifice, and then, in mid-sacrifice, achieve emotional Zen by realizing this is no sacrifice at all. Not many people have true, conditional love. It is easier to skip work and pretend the love is unconditional. But that's not love. That's just ignoring the bills. KT, you never ignore the bills. I won't either.

Thank you to my family for unconditional love. Thank you to Mom and Dad for being the only people sitting in that court room on one of the worst days of my life. To Joe for the role model. To AJ for the friendship. To Katie for really wanting to see me. And to my kids, who have given my life real meaning. What I think about most often when I'm running is my family, our pasts, present, and future. You mean the world to me.

Thank you to Ryan Varga and Ben Spann who read early drafts of this book and gave me permission to believe in it.

Thank you to Sophie Sunny, who caught hundreds of errors even after I'd proofread the manuscript myself several times. I'm nervous adding these words right now because you won't have the chance to fix spelling, to add the comma I always forget in a list of three things and to make this book look like it was written by someone who know how to write.

Thank you to all the amateur runners who encourage others.

Books, podcasts, and social media have all been friends on my running journey. People helping people is the flow of love, of hope and bravery, of vulnerability and strength. This includes Professor Katy Milkman from the opening chapter.

Lastly, thank you to everyone who reads and shares this book. The recommendation of a friend is a powerful gift, and I'm honored to be a tiny piece of that generosity.

References

This is a list of works and people to whom my running owes a lot. However, they're not personal relationships. Any reader of this book can access this list and improve their life. I'm grateful for the difference this list made for me, and feel it is my responsibility to pass it along.

Podcasts
- *The Running Explained Podcast* w/ Elisabeth Scott
- *The Strength Running Podcast* w/ Jason Fitzgerald
- *The Nick Bare Podcast*
- *The Run Smarter Podcast* w/ Brodie Sharpe
- *Marathon Training Academy* w/ Angie and Trevor
- *The Jeremy Miller Podcast*

I've listened to hundreds of hours of these podcasts. I often found myself stopping, texting myself a note, and being launched into new realms of research and learning that has helped me improve my relationship with my body and with running. Every one of them is a wealth of knowledge.

Audiobooks
- *How to Lose a Marathon* by Joel Cohen
- *My Year of Running Dangerously* by Tom Foreman
- *What I Talk About When I Talk About Running* by Haruki Murakami
- *Running with the Buffaloes* by Chris Lear

- *Running to the Edge* by Matthew Futterman
- *26 Marathons* by Meb Keflezighi
- *Iron War* by Matt Fitzgerald
- *Can't Hurt Me* by David Goggins
- *Endure* by Cam Hanes
- *Born to Run* by Christopher McDougall
- *North* by Scott & Jenny Jurek
- *Running to the Edge* by Matthew Futterman

There are a lot of running books, but these were my favorite. McDougall's *Born to Run* was my entry into running books, and Murakami's memoir is my personal favorite, but each of these found a special place in my heart. I owe a special thanks to Tom Foreman's *My Year of Running Dangerously* for its humor and relatability letting me realize my running notes could become a book. The quality of Foreman's storytelling is inspirational (and maybe the funniest book on the list. No worse than second funniest behind Cohen, who wrote for The Simpsons).

Websites
- RunnersWorld.com
- RunToTheFinish.com
- PrecisionHydration.com
- FindMyMarathon.com

Run to the Finish by Amanda Brooks was great guidance for an amateur. Runner's World is the mecca. The only website I routinely tell people about is PrecisionHydration.com. It is the very best resource I've found to understand what your body needs for distance training. I learned of it after the Disney Marathon, and it made a massive impact on my long runs and led directly to a new marathon PR in my next effort. I will provide a primer of those hydration and fueling lessons in the amendment that follows these references. As for FindMyMarathon.com, it has fantastic stats to help you know what to expect from a course, and if you're thinking of running a full marathon, it's my favorite site for help in making a selection of which race is good for you.

Instagram & Social Media Personalities
- Matt Choi - @mattchoi_6
- Jeremy Miller - @jeremymille.r
- David Goggins - @davidgoggins
- Amanda Brooks - @runtothefinish
- Squat University - @squat_university
- Meg Takacs - @meg_takacs
- Nick Bare - @nickbarefitness

My favorite social media accounts are the ones that make me want to put social media down and get moving. Huge shouts to Jeremy Miller and Matt Choi specifically. They're strong runners, but not elite. They're two amateurs who got into content creation and really opened my eyes to the daily life of running. They're larger accounts now, but Jeremy specifically had less than five thousand followers when I found him, and I can say his methodology hasn't changed too radically. They're both great examples of what a huge impact the dedication to running can have on an individual's life and the community of people that individual supports.

Amendment: Hydration

During the Disney Marathon, I was woefully uneducated on proper hydration. What I discovered while training for my next marathon was that I needed far more salt. Instead of telling you a story, I'll just give you a quick primer on the topic here so that you can start experimenting and building your own fuel and hydration plans.

There are three intakes you need to think about before & during running:

- Carbs (glycogen)
- Salt (electrolytes)
- Fluid

If you run too low on any of these you will hit the wall (cramp/bonk/crash/explode). Most people have enough stored resources for about 60-120 minutes of continuous exercise. Running is one of humanity's most efficient movements, so it's typically closer to the 12 0minute side, but there's a lot of reasons to dial your numbers in on shorter runs too. Benefits of proper fueling and hydration for any workouts are:

- Feel less fatigued
- Prevent cramps
- Recover faster
- Train at higher intensity

- Feel less sleepy post-run

The best resource I've found on this topic is PrecisionHydration.com. Their Knowledge Hub is excellent, and I recommend everyone go take the free fueling quiz. It will generate an initial plan for your personal fuel and hydration needs. Here's the numbers from my initial plan for my last marathon (intake is per hour):

- Carbs – 60g
- Sodium – 1500mg per 32oz
- Fluid – 15oz

After testing throughout my training, I realized I felt better at higher doses, so I increased my intakes slightly. Eventually I settled on a plan for my next marathon. Every hour I filled an eighteen ounce running bottle with one Maurten Drink Mix and a packet of LMNT electrolytes. I took a Maurten Gel every thirty minutes (using the caffeine gel every other time), and took that gel with two ounces of water at an aid station which bumped up my fluid intake and diluted my sodium ratio. Bottom line, my in-race fueling and hydration numbers per hour looked like this for the San Antonio Marathon:

- Carbs - 90g
- Sodium - 2,100mg per 32oz
- Fluid - 22oz

The danger is too much carbs and sodium can give you the shits or stomach cramps. Too much fluid and you have to pee. Start on the lower end and work up to the amount you need. Here's my fav sources of each.

Carbs:
1. **Drink Mix** - All you need for shorter runs. Blends easily with your fluid and offers additional sodium. My favorites are 1) Maurten 2) Tailwind 3) G1M Sport
2. **Gels** - Easiest to store and digest. They have no fluid and are usually lower in sodium than the drink mix. My favorites are 1) Maurten 2) GU 3) Spring
3. **Chews/Stroopwafel** – In my opinion, these are only for people who hate gels or need variation. These options have less carb density and are harder to store, but check them out if you hate gels.

Sodium/Electrolytes:
*Note: What you use for carbs will inform how much sodium you need from these products.

On sodium, the important part is concentration. Drinking water dilutes the electrolyte volume in your blood, so your heart pushes less electrolytes to the muscle with each beat. That's often why your heart is beating so hard; it's just going as fast as it needs to for your muscle to have its full supply of resources. Yes, that's oxygen, but it's also electrolytes. By adding enough salt and not too much water, you increase the volume of sodium in your blood, so your heart needn't work as hard, and you can both run longer and recover faster.

1. **Drink Powders:**
o   LMNT - My fav, but only comes in 1,000mg per 16oz packets, so requires a little extra work
o   BPN Electrolytes - Comes in a tub, so it's easier to manipulate how much you want.
2. **Salt Pills/Chews** - Great tack-on, usually about 250mg you can carry with you and take as needed.
3. **Gatorade** - only mentioning because it's usually the only salt

you'll find on many race courses. If it's super hot or you're getting a bit crampy, always select the Gatorade at aid stations, not the water.

Fluid
1. **Water** – The only water I would use on the course is what I blend with my drink mix and electrolytes in my water bottle, and the water I take with my gels. That said, you could take Gatorade with your gels if you want to err on more electrolytes and carbs than less. If you haven't refilled a water bottle on a course before, just run to the backside of the aid station and fill straight from the cooler into your bottle. It's a common and accepted practice.

One more thing—Pre-loading electrolytes:
If I'm running for over an hour, I like to preload. For me, that's 500-1500mg sodium in 16oz of water. The longer I'm going to be running, the denser I'll make my 16oz solution. I will eat at least 60g of carbs (oatmeal, pasta, fruit, etc). This aids in all the benefits outlined earlier.

If it's a half or marathon race day where I'm not just running long but also at full intensity, I will drink a 1,500mg per 16oz the night before and increase the pre-race load to 2,000-3,000mg per 16oz. I'll also double the carbs and give myself a 90-minute digestion window.

Experiment early and find what feels food for you.

Epilogue
The San Antonio Marathon

I feel the faint, mile-marking buzz on my wrist and look at my watch. Mile twenty is finished. I've been running for three hours, four minutes, and fifty seconds. Pace is 9:08 per mile. The four-hour marathon pace is 9:09. Devoid of context, I'm perfectly on track to run my first sub-four-hour marathon.

Unfortunately, I'm drowning in context.

Four miles ago, the faint buzz on my wrist showed me 8:59 per mile. I felt a familiar "whoopsie" in my hamstring in mile sixteen, and my body has been breaking down ever since. Miles seventeen to twenty clocked in at 10:04, 9:54, 10:37, and 10:23. I've been here before. The hamstrings dried out like jerky, the battery-acid blood, and the bone-on-bone crunch in my ankles are all signs that I am finished. The tank is empty. And yet, if I am to achieve my goal, I must run for one more hour at nine-minute miles. I haven't run a nine-minute mile since Mile 14. That was more than an hour ago.

Hope is dim, and yet, hope is there. I *have* been here before, but I don't feel the anxiety of failure like I did before. Instead, a scene from *Mad Men* enters my heart, and I hear Don Draper saying, "In Greek, nostalgia literally means 'the pain from an old wound.' It's a twinge in your heart far more powerful than memory alone." Yes, that's what this is. I thought the tank was empty, but it's not. Down in the bottom of the reservoir is experience that gives me certainty. Suffering at mile 20, I am exactly where I intended. I pick up the pace. And I have a thought that makes me smile.

At least I haven't shit my pants.

I finished the San Antonio Marathon before I finalized the manuscript of *Looks Like We're Running*. It's the race I'm most proud of to-date, not just because of the race, but because of the training that went into it. I avoided injury, I ran several fifty-mile weeks, and I incorporated far better practices around fuel and hydration. Still, I don't know if there are extra lessons. I think perhaps there's just routine transformation—perhaps distortion—as I persist within the running process. It is a process that has both enriched me and lessened me, like a blade that is sharper because it's been ground down. Grinding myself through the miles used to seem like sacrifice. Now the hardship of the miles feels hygenic and meditative. They grind away my ego, and I can see myself more clearly.

In many ways, *Looks Like We're Running* is my offer to others, a sales pitch for why they should run, even if they can't do it well (*especially* if they can't do it well). Perhaps I've failed to explain the true lure, and if I have, let me offer one final articulation from someone who wrote it better than I can. I read Matt Fitzgerald's *Iron War* a few months after San Antonio, and in it, he perfectly describes the ultimate promise of distance training:

In the hardest moments of a long race, the athlete's entire conscious experience of reality boils down to a desire to continue pitted against a desire to quit. Nothing else remains. The athlete is no longer a student or a teacher or a salesman. He is no longer a son or a father or a husband. He has no social roles or human connections whatsoever. He is utterly alone. He no longer has any possessions. There is no yesterday and no tomorrow, only now. The agony of extreme endurance fatigue crowds out every thought and feeling except one: the goal of reaching the finish line. The sensations within the body—burning lungs, screaming muscles, whole-body enervation—exist only as the substance of the desire to quit. What little of the external environment the athlete is aware of

—the road ahead, the competitor behind, the urgings of onlookers—exists only as the substance of the desire to continue. The desire to continue versus the desire to quit—the athlete is this and this alone until he chooses one or the other. And when the choice is made he briefly becomes either persevering or quitting until, after he has stopped at the finish line or, God forbid, short of it, the stripped-away layers are piled back on and he becomes his old self again. Only not quite. He is changed, for better or worse.

A book has to be finished at some point, so this post-credits scene is the last pitch. That quote from *Iron War* is the final offer. Maybe stripping away so many layers sounds awful right now, but sit with it. The process of life distorts both us and the ideas we're offered. Like a Don Draper quote, you might be surprised when you find it useful.

Mile seventeen in San Antonio is the first ten-minue mile of the race. I make a choice. I consume every bit of fuel I have on my person. Every salt tablet, electrolyte powder and sugary gel goes into my system immediately. This is my only recourse against the dehydration and cramps beginning to surface. If all that fuel prevents cramps, why didn't I take it sooner? Well, the downside of too much sodium is incontinence. If you follow endurance sports, seeing athletes urinate or defecate on themselves is not uncommon. So as I take in nearly 3,000mg of salt with very little fluid on top of everything else I'd ingested during the race, I am nervous. Still, I have to know that I'm doing all I can, that I'm giving it my best effort. I'll either shit my pants, or I'll give sub-four hours my absolute best effort. Maybe both. Over the next three miles, I burn my time margin to let the fuel get into my system while I run at a triage pace. Now, there are 6.2 miles to go and a lot of pain in front of me, but at least I haven't shit my pants.

Can I run 6.2 miles in fifty-five minutes? I've done it several times. It's a 10K. My fastest 10K ever was forty-six minutes and twenty-one seconds. I tell myself my body has it. I tell myself the only thing limiting me is my mind. I tell myself that fatigue is a trick of the body, and cramps are neurological fraud. I also tell myself to pace it. Mile twenty-one is 9:17.

Pace it a little faster. Mile twenty-two is 9:07.

Mile twenty-three starts off with a half-mile uphill. On the way down, I try to make up time, and my hamstring seizes. This latest argument against neurological fraud is compelling. Mile twenty-three is a 9:37. I hobble, stop, and order myself a ten count. *One... two...three...*I remember the Chicago Marathon, where stretching a cramp gave me nearly twenty minutes of redemption. It was enough then to look like I was running to the only spectator who cared. *Four...five...six...*If I can look like I'm running for twenty minutes now, I'll be in the last mile. Then it's just a mile. I can always push for a mile. *Seven...eight...nine...* Go get it.

Mile twenty-four is 8:42.

My right hamstring cramps, so I stop kicking it back and start swinging it out to the side of me like a peg leg so I barely have to bend the knee. It's more work, but as long as I can not cramp, I can push. Mile twenty-five is 8:43.

My left calf is cramping, presumably from the extra work incurred in the peg-leg style. I push off the heel for relief. I no longer look like I'm running, but I look at my watch, and the pace says 9:11. I try to do math. Two seconds times twenty-six miles, that's less than a minute, right? I'm so close. If I can just find a way to move my body for an eight-minute mile, I might do it. My heart rate is maxed out. My skin feels like it's fire-engine red. Every step is a negotiation with screaming joints and comatose muscles. But somehow, it's working. Mile twenty-six is 8:07.

The pace on my watch says 9:09! I'm so close. I'm suddenly aware of all the abstract visions that have been driving me for the last six miles. My kids. My wife. My brothers and sister. It all kind of collides into a vision of myself, my inner hero. I funnel this hero directly against the clock, hobbling furiously towards the finish line. I'm over the line! It's done. Thank God it's done. I limp over to the side of the finishing zone, the shortest distance to be at a complete stop. I force myself to stand erect and both quads immediately cramp up. I buckle, my hands go to my knees. Someone runs over and asks if I need medical. I try to smile and say, "Maybe six miles ago." They hand me a Gatorade and leave me alone.

Briefly, I feel a moment of nothingness, then I notice the salt caking in the crow's feet of my eyes. I'm squinting at a sign with a QR code offering my official time. *My time!* I stop my watch at 4:01:14. Had it been over a minute since I crossed the line? I try to think of the starting line. Did I begin the watch timer a little early or a little late? Not that it matters. Despite my frantic attachment to my watch's data, the watch is not the clock I killed myself for over the last hour. I need the official time. My back barely pulls me off my knees. My feet are screaming. My toes throb. Was I really running only a couple minutes ago? I shuffle towards the sign.

I scan the code.

I type my last name.

Official time, 4:00:36.

Printed in the USA
CPSIA information can be obtained
at www.ICGtesting.com
LVHW040727251023
762015LV00002B/7